THE WHICH? GUIDE TO
CHILDREN'S HEALTH

About the contributors

Contributing editor:
Dr Harry Brown, full-time GP

Other contributors:
Dr Steve Conway, consultant physician and paediatrician and senior clinical lecturer in the Department of Paediatrics and Child Health at the University of Leeds

Sophie Kay, paediatric community nurse, with several years' experience as a health visitor

Dr David Moore, full-time GP

Dr Adrian Mullish, dental practitioner

Dr Kenneth Shenderey, full-time GP

The Editor and Publishers would also like to thank the British Red Cross; Sue Wolfe, chief paediatric dietitian at St James's and Seacroft University Hospitals NHS Trust, Leeds; and the Research Council for Complementary Medicine; also Clara Baloyi, Jane Chumbley, David Friedman and Marie Lorimer

THE WHICH? GUIDE TO CHILDREN'S HEALTH

EDITOR: DR HARRY BROWN

CONSUMERS' ASSOCIATION

Which? Books are commissioned and researched by
Consumers' Association and published by
Which? Ltd, 2 Marylebone Road, London NW1 4DF
email address: guide.reports@which.net

Distributed by The Penguin Group:
Penguin Books Ltd, 27 Wrights Lane, London W8 5TZ

First edition September 1997
Copyright © 1997 Which? Ltd

British Library Cataloguing-in-Publication Data
A catalogue record for this book is available from the British Library

ISBN 0 85202 655 2

For a full list of Which? books, please write to Which? Books, Castlemead,
Gascoyne Way, Hertford X, SG14 1LH, or access our web site at
http://www.which.net

Typographic design by Paul Saunders
Cover design by Ridgeway Associates
Cover photograph by Tony Stone Images
Typeset by Saxon Graphics Ltd, Derby
Printed in England by Clays Ltd, St Ives plc

CONTENTS

INTRODUCTION 7

1 BEFORE THE BIRTH OF YOUR BABY 9

2 YOUR NEWBORN BABY AND THE FIRST YEAR 15

3 GETTING YOUR CHILD IMMUNISED 42

4 YOUR CHILD'S HEALTH AND DEVELOPMENT 53

5 A GUIDE TO SENSIBLE EATING 91

6 BEHAVIOURAL AND EMOTIONAL PROBLEMS 109

7 CARE OF YOUR CHILD'S TEETH 123

8 GETTING THE BEST MEDICAL CARE FOR YOUR CHILD 133

9 AN A–Z OF ILLNESSES AND SYMPTOMS 146

10 ACCIDENT PREVENTION AND FIRST AID 251

ADDRESSES★ 272

INDEX 275

★ An asterisk next to the name of an organisation in the text indicates that the address can be found in this section

INTRODUCTION

Children born in Britain at the dawn of the new millennium can in many ways be regarded as fortunate. Only a couple of generations ago, outbreaks of infectious diseases such as whooping cough and measles were all too common and often claimed lives, diphtheria and tuberculosis remained a widespread threat and poliomyelitis crippled thousands.

Since that time, advances in medicine – immunisation and screening programmes, better drugs, more sophisticated therapies and surgical treatment – and improved living conditions have helped to provide a safer world and to reduce infant mortality. On the other hand, new problems have arisen, including air pollution, ever-growing traffic volumes which have made our streets unsafe for children and the advent of disorders such as anorexia that were unheard of in the earlier post-war years, together with our growing awareness of the adverse effects that allergies and food intolerances can have upon health. None of these issues makes the role of a parent any easier.

What all parents can do, however, is to ensure that they give their children the best possible start in life, and to be aware of the problems that can arise. Most children develop into adults with few health problems, but during the years of childhood their parents will from time to time want to know the answers to a multitude of questions relating to their health and development.

These might include some of the controversial topics of recent years, such as how to avoid the risk of cot death, or issues on which medical advice has changed radically over the few decades (such as the practice of removing tonsils and adenoids, which is therefore not covered in this book). Or they might be specific queries of the type that follow:

- How can I be sure that my baby is getting enough milk?

- Is it really worthwhile vaccinating my baby when some of the immunisations themselves carry risks?
- How can I encourage my child into a good sleeping routine?
- My child seems to have a constant cough: could he have asthma?
- What is the difference between a fit and a faint?
- How can I best help my child to have good teeth?

All the health professionals involved in the book have first-hand experience of answering just this sort of question, and all are parents. Their starting point was that although there is no substitute for seeking proper medical advice, it is often helpful to read about an illness or a problem in the calm of your home; also, it is reassuring to have on hand a guide to help you decide what to do when your child becomes ill, thereby perhaps preventing a small problem escalating into a crisis: does this symptom call for urgent action? should I wait before taking my child to the doctor? what else can I do in the meantime or in the long term?

Decisions that you may need to take before the birth of your baby, dental matters, normal childhood development and emotional and behavioural problems are all discussed, in addition to worries that tend to crop up in the first year and the familiar childhood illnesses. Where appropriate, the use of complementary therapies is considered. Many of the illnesses and symptoms appear in the A-Z that starts on page 146, but consult the index if you cannot immediately find a subject. The book also contains information about basic first aid (page 251) and helps you get the best for your family from the health service.

The guide does not claim to be encyclopaedic but on the other hand some unusual conditions are included for good reasons. For example, brain tumours and meningitis are both very rare, yet many a parent taking a child with a headache to see the doctor asks if these conditions might be the cause of the problem. Equally, infectious diseases that are now rare, such as whooping cough and measles, are covered in order to show why it is important to immunise against them.

You cannot take your child's health for granted. This book is full of information and practical advice on how to maximise your child's health – one of the most important things that you can do for him or her.

CHAPTER 1

BEFORE THE BIRTH OF YOUR BABY

ALL parents are concerned for the health of their children. From the minute they are born, parents have a responsibility for their children's wellbeing, but caring for a child actually begins well before birth. In fact, the future health of your precious baby may be affected by factors even before conception.

There is a great deal that a prospective mother can do to ensure that her baby has the best possible start in life, starting by optimising her own health and treating any pre-existing medical problems.

Stopping smoking

Everyone knows that smoking is bad for health in a multitude of ways and yet plenty of people still smoke. However, knowing that smoking is going to affect the health of your newborn baby may be a more persuasive argument. Smoking can impede a baby's growth in the womb, and the incidence of miscarriage, premature births and stillbirths may be higher in pregnant smokers.

It will help you if your partner gives up smoking at the same time. Apart from providing moral support, it lessens the risks of passive smoking. It is important to stop smoking before conception rather than in the first few weeks of pregnancy, as early pregnancy is a critical period in the development of a baby and smoking will adversely affect the growing embryo. Remember, it may be a few weeks before you find out that you are pregnant.

Giving up smoking is easier said than done – more often than not, willpower is the critical factor. However, some people find hypnosis or acupuncture helpful.

Giving up or reducing alcohol intake

It is important to recognise that alcohol is a drug and that like all drugs it poses a danger to a growing embryo in the womb. In fact, excess alcohol intake during pregnancy can lead to a specific disease called Foetal Alcohol Syndrome. This can cause multiple abnormalities in the baby, including brain damage, which can result in severe learning difficulties. It is not known what constitutes a safe level of alcohol intake, so you might decide to avoid it altogether.

However, guidelines have been issued by the Royal College of Obstetricians and Gynaecologists stating that no proven detrimental effect has been observed in an unborn baby in terms of growth or IQ if the mother consumes less than 15 units of alcohol a week. (One unit of alcohol equates roughly to a small glass of wine or a single measure of spirits.)

Discuss with your doctor any concerns about your alcohol intake before or during pregnancy, and get your partner to reduce or eliminate his own intake to support you.

Limiting drugs

After the thalidomide tragedy of the 1960s everyone became aware of the dangers to unborn children of both prescribed and over-the-counter medicines. All drugs – whether legal or illegal – should be treated as being potentially dangerous and harmful to the unborn baby. This principle should also be borne in mind during the time you are trying to conceive. Always remind your doctor – and your dentist – that you are pregnant when he or she writes a prescription for you. Don't assume that they will remember and even if they are aware you are pregnant, seek specific reassurance that the drug prescribed is both appropriate and safe during pregnancy. If you are in doubt, confirm with the pharmacist when the prescription is being dispensed. Very few drugs are known to be completely safe during pregnancy.

If you are taking any regular medication or suffer from a chronic condition such as diabetes or epilepsy, the therapy or disease could have a bearing on the health of your unborn baby. It is important to discuss with your doctor *prior* to becoming pregnant how your condition will be affected by pregnancy.

Reviewing what you eat

Pregnant women should eat a healthy balanced diet consisting of sensible amounts of carbohydrates, fat, protein, vitamins and minerals. Minimise your intake of junk foods and reduce caffeine by cutting down on tea, coffee and cola drinks. Dieting during pregnancy is not wise – what you store in your reserves may also be utilised by a growing baby.

Exercise

Take moderate amounts of gentle exercise – walking and swimming are ideal – interspersed by plenty of rest. Exercise classes should take into account the fact that you are pregnant.

Boosting folic acid

All women planning a pregnancy should take a supplement of 400 micrograms of folic acid a day from the moment they begin trying to conceive. They should continue taking supplements of this vitamin until the pregnancy is at least 12 weeks advanced. This action has been shown to reduce the incidence of spina bifida. If a previous child has been affected by spina bifida, then the dose should be increased to 5 milligrams of folic acid a day. Tablets containing the necessary 400-microgram supplements are available from chemists without the need for a prescription.

Infections harmful to the newborn baby

There are a multitude of infections that can cause damage to a growing baby in the womb. Some are worth mentioning in specific detail but if you are exposed to any infectious illness, it is always worth checking with your doctor.

Sexually transmitted diseases

Gonorrhoea, genital herpes, syphilis and AIDS are significant diseases which can be sexually transmitted, although there are other routes of entry, apart from sexual intercourse, for the AIDS virus to infiltrate the body. If there is any possibility, no matter how remote, that you as a prospective mother may be at risk of such a disease, then a visit to a genito-urinary clinic or your GP is strongly advised.

Rubella

Also known as German measles, this causes a relatively trivial illness in the mother but can have devastating consequences – deafness, heart defects, brain damage – for her unborn baby, particularly if it occurs in early pregnancy. This is wholly preventable by making sure that the mother has been immunised. Even so, all women contemplating pregnancy should have a blood test to confirm that they are still immune so that immunisation can be offered if necessary.

Cytomegalovirus

This is a relatively common infectious hazard to a baby in the womb and occurs in 3 out of 1,000 live births. Infections in early pregnancy can cause a miscarriage, and learning disabilities, epilepsy and deafness in babies who survive. Like rubella, cytomegalovirus can cause a minor illness in adults, or can cause a disorder similar to glandular fever, but it is often asymptomatic and the adult is not even aware of it. However, unlike rubella, there is currently no reliable vaccine.

Toxoplasmosis

Toxoplasmosis has gained notoriety because it can be caught through handling cat's faeces, as well as undercooked or raw meat. If you discover that you are pregnant take precautions: get someone else to clear out the cat's litter tray, wear gloves for gardening and wash your hands after touching soil in order to avoid coming into contact with cat's droppings. Toxoplasmosis can cause brain damage in the baby while the mother suffers merely a mild, often asymptomatic, version of the illness.

Listeria
A rare but important cause of serious problems in a newborn baby, listeria can also cause stillbirth. The organism *Listeria monocytogenes* has a remarkable ability to survive in adverse conditions such as low temperatures, so make sure you thoroughly reheat cook-chill meals and avoid all types of pâté, and soft ripened cheeses such as Camembert and Brie as well as blue-veined types.

Genetic screening

The word 'congenital' means present at birth and is often used to describe an abnormality or defect in a newborn baby. The specific causes of a congenital abnormality are usually not precisely known, but may occur through both genetic and environmental influences. Occasionally, an abnormality may be caused by a specific genetic defect, as in the case of Down's Syndrome, or by exposure to some harmful substance that affects the growing baby, as in the thalidomide cases; or there is a contribution from both the genes and the baby's (and mother's) environment.

Our unique genetic make-up is governed by codes within the DNA which lies at the centre of cells in our bodies. The characteristics of DNA are passed down from our parents. The presence of some genes indicates a propensity to develop certain diseases in later life. If certain diseases run in families an abnormal or rogue gene is usually responsible. Means of identifying these abnormal genes are now being found, and carriers for the particular condition as well those who are actually affected can be identified. This means that if a condition runs in a family it may be possible for the pregnant woman to have her foetus tested.

This has important implications for the woman and her partner. If she agrees to a screening test, of whatever nature, she has to understand the full ramifications of a positive or a negative result. In particular, she should ask herself: if she knew that she was carrying a baby with a particular condition would she terminate the pregnancy?

Remember also that performing some tests may in itself pose a possible hazard to the unborn child. Before being offered any test of this nature, it is essential to have proper counselling.

Amniocentesis

This involves extracting a sample of the amniotic fluid that surrounds the baby in the womb. A number of genetic conditions such as Down's Syndrome can be diagnosed from the sample. The procedure is usually performed at 14-20 weeks of pregnancy: first an ultrasound scan is performed to check the position of both the baby and the placenta; the sample is then sucked out via a needle inserted through the tummy wall. The results can take up to a fortnight to be conveyed to the parents and the procedure is not without risk. It can cause damage to the baby or the placenta and the miscarriage rate is about 1 per cent.

Chorionic villus biopsy

This involves taking a sample of the developing placenta either through the tummy wall or via the vagina. It is an alternative to amniocentesis, capable of showing up the same range of problems, and can be performed about 9-11 weeks into the pregnancy. However, there may be a higher risk of miscarriage compared to amniocentesis.

Triple or quadruple blood test

This is a test of substances which are found in the bloodstream of a pregnant woman. The tests indicate only a probability of the baby having Down's Syndrome and further tests such as amniocentesis may be necessary.

Complementary therapies in pregnancy and labour

As with conventional medicine, it is wise to avoid all therapies unless prescribed by a qualified practitioner. Even then, use a therapy known to be safe in pregnancy only under expert supervision and when the symptoms experienced are intolerable. Herbal medicines, acupressure and aromatherapy have been used in the treatment of morning sickness and heartburn, and massage and hypnosis for anxiety. During labour, hypnosis, massage, acupuncture and aromatherapy have all been used successfully in the management of pain relief.

CHAPTER 2

YOUR NEWBORN BABY AND THE FIRST YEAR

WHETHER you plan to have your baby at home or in a hospital maternity unit, your baby will be monitored during labour and delivery. If all has gone well during the pregnancy the only healthcare professional involved in your care may be your midwife.

If the birth is to take place at home your community midwife will look after you, but be sure to ask for identification if your usual midwife is otherwise engaged and another midwife not known to you is standing in. Hospital maternity units and labour wards have their own midwives, but some units allow, and even encourage, your own community midwife to continue to care for you during your labour and delivery in the hospital.

Problems may occur during labour that the midwife feels warrant the presence and opinion of a doctor. At home this could be your own GP or one of the partners in the practice; in hospital it would be one of the doctors working in the maternity unit. Additionally, a doctor specialising in the care of children – a paediatrician – may be asked to attend. The paediatrician will have the necessary equipment and expertise to care for the newborn baby if any problems arise.

During labour or delivery, you may be asked if student midwives or student doctors could be present, observing and possibly assisting in your care. They would be closely monitored by qualified staff but you have every right to refuse permission. Your care should not be influenced in any way by your decision. Remember, however, that all qualified midwives and doctors started their careers as students.

Problems with your baby during or after delivery may be anticipated or may come out of the blue; if you are at home you may have to be transferred to hospital. Problems that are anticipated can be prepared for by having the staff and equipment ready and waiting as labour progresses. This usually means having your baby in a hospital which has a specialised intensive care unit, often known as SCBU (Special Care Baby Unit) or NNU (Neonatal Unit). Within the NHS, there are only a certain number of intensive care beds. At any particular time your local unit may be full, so you may have to travel to another unit, perhaps in another city, to give birth or have your baby cared for after delivery.

For the first ten days after the birth of the baby a midwife will visit the mother and baby at home to check on both of them and to offer advice on feeding, bathing and any other matters that may be of concern to the mother.

The first minutes of life

Every parent is overjoyed when the newborn baby first cries. The first few seconds waiting for this to happen can seem an eternity. A baby may sometimes need a little help to start off the process of breathing. Fluids may be cleared from the baby's lungs by the use of a simple suction tube, and a cool jet of oxygen may be blown over the baby's nose to stimulate respiration. Once the baby is breathing and becoming 'pink' he or she will be wrapped in a warm towel and given back to the mother.

Usually at this point it is likely that you will be offered a vitamin K injection for your baby. This injection can prevent bleeding problems straight after birth, particularly in the brain. The evidence for its efficacy is pretty strong but it would be sensible to discuss the matter with your obstetrician before you go into labour.

If a baby does not start breathing, or if an initially happy and apparently well baby becomes distressed, he or she will be transferred to the neonatal unit, a high-tech ward full of machines, wires and electronic displays. These may trigger anxiety, but the trained staff will explain their purpose and how they can help your baby get off to a good start.

Premature babies

The majority of babies born at 37 weeks or later are healthy and adapt to their new way of life without any problems. Before 37 weeks, however, a baby is said to be premature, or pre-term. Pre-term labour occurs more often in first pregnancies, teenage mothers and those mothers who have had certain conditions and illnesses during pregnancy. This can bring along a number of problems in the neonatal (newborn) period. The survival rates of premature babies are improving all the time because of the advances in care at the specialised neonatal units. More and more babies born as early as 24 to 28 weeks or as light as 1 kg are now surviving.

The main question now is how far to go. It is known that parent–child bonding can be interfered with by the separation caused by the necessary treatments in a neonatal unit. There also seems to be an increase in cot death and child abuse in these children.

The problems associated with prematurity are numerous; the more common complications follow. However, it is important to remember that perfectly normal children can develop from very premature babies who have had a stormy introduction to life.

- **Brain damage** Pre-term babies, particularly very premature ones, are at risk of brain haemorrhages, possibly due to oxygen starvation. About 1 in 5 of babies who weigh less than 1.5kg at birth may have bleeding in their brain. This can be demonstrated by scans performed shortly after birth. Many babies will not show any symptoms though some will have periods when they stop breathing or become very floppy. These infants are at high risk of developing brain damage and may develop conditions such as cerebral palsy.
- **Feeding** A premature baby may find the effort of suckling too much, so milk and supplements will be given by a fine plastic tube passed down through one of the baby's nostrils into the back of the throat and down into the stomach. In some cases it is possible for expressed breast milk to be given by this method.

- **Temperature regulation** Premature babies lose heat very rapidly, so neonatal units provide a controlled temperature either in an incubator or by using radiant heaters.
- **Breathing** Most but not all premature babies have immature lungs and air passages. This can lead to breathing difficulties, the so-called Respiratory Distress Syndrome. Fluids sucked into the baby's lungs before, during or after delivery may add to this problem. The symptoms may range from mild changes in the rate of breathing for a few days, through to severe breathing difficulties with added complications and, unfortunately in some cases, death. Respiratory distress is managed in a neonatal unit and involves considerable medical and nursing expertise. X-ray pictures may be taken and the baby may need help with breathing by the use of a machine called a ventilator. An intravenous line or 'drip' may be needed to give the baby vital fluids and medicines.
- **Infection** Premature babies have weakened defence systems and are therefore more susceptible to infections. The common infections attack the chest, bowel and urinary system. However, these infections can quickly pass into the bloodstream resulting in septicaemia, or cause meningitis – inflammation of the tissues which line the brain and spinal cord. Treatment with antibiotics and other drugs is usually required.

Low birth-weight babies

A baby born at term or even an overdue baby may be affected by the same problems that may be encountered by a premature baby, particularly if it is of low birth weight, for whatever reason.

The examination of the newborn baby

From the minute the baby is born, the midwife will observe the baby and watch out for any problems. For example, she will make sure that the baby is breathing properly and that there are no obvious abnormalities. It is likely that in the 24 hours following birth a paediatrician will give the baby a complete check-up. If possible the examination will be done in the presence of the mother to give her the opportunity to ask any questions. This check will be repeated at six weeks, probably by the GP.

What the doctor is looking for

- **Skin** – skin blemishes and jaundice.
- **Head** – the fontanelles (the soft spots in the skull) will be felt and the general shape of the skull assessed. The paediatrician will put a finger inside the baby's mouth to make sure the palate is fully formed. Although it is difficult to examine the functioning of the baby's brain, he or she will observe the baby's general behaviour and responses. The eyes are examined in particular to check for the (uncommon) condition of congenital cataracts.
- **Chest** – in addition to watching the baby's breathing pattern, the doctor will listen to the chest as well as the heart, particularly to make sure there are no heart murmurs. A heart murmur is a vibration from an unusually turbulent flow of blood through the heart; this may (or may not) be the first indication of a heart defect.
- **Tummy** – as a matter of routine the tummy will be felt in order to detect any lumps or bumps and make sure that vital organs such as the liver, kidneys and spleen are not enlarged. The doctor will also have a look at the back passage to make sure that the anus is normally formed and to see if the baby has passed its first meconium, which is the thick, greeny-black stools normally passed in the first day or so of life. (During labour, meconium can be passed through the birth canal; this can be a sign that the baby is in some form of distress and that medical attention may be needed.) Once feeding is started, meconium is replaced by normal bowel motions. Failure to pass meconium may imply that the bowels have not formed properly or that there is an abnormal narrowing within a section of the bowel.
- **Spine** – the doctor will check that the spine is normally formed and will make sure that no spina bifida is present.
- **Genitals** – the doctor will examine the baby boy's testicles and ensure that they have descended. If they have not, they should be re-examined at regular intervals over the next few months. Abnormalities of the penis are self-evident – see pages 37–9. Occasionally, the breast of both boys and girls will be enlarged and may even produce drops of milk. This is known as witch's milk but it has an entirely innocent explanation – the mother's

hormones are crossing the placenta and acting on the baby. This phenomenon will soon disappear as the hormones are chemically destroyed by the baby.

- **Groin** – babies (more boys than girls) are sometimes born with an inguinal hernia, a bulge from the groin that may contain loops of bowel. An operation to repair it is likely to be required.

- **Hips** – congenital dislocation of the hip is an important condition for doctors to search for and exclude. If present, it means that the head of the thigh bone – the femur – does not fit properly into its socket in the pelvis. Failure of the head of the femur to locate properly in the pelvis will mean that the hip will easily dislocate. If left untreated the hip will not develop properly and as a result the child could develop a limp when learning to walk. In future years the child may be at risk of developing a prematurely arthritic hip. The cause is unclear but the incidence is about 1 in 800 children.

  Children at high risk of congenital dislocation of the hip include those born in the extended breech position as well as those with a family history of the condition.

  There is a test for this condition which all newborn babies should undergo. The baby is placed on his or her back and the knees are bent. The hips are swivelled outwards so that the knees are almost flat against the table. If the joint is abnormal a clunk may be heard. This manoeuvre can be repeated to confirm the findings. This procedure should be carried out only by a trained medical person and should not be attempted by parents.

  If congenital dislocation of the hip is identified, the hips are splinted. The splint is applied to both hips equally, keeping the thighs bent and the legs splayed outwards. All affected babies should be referred to an orthopaedic specialist.

- **Hands and feet** – a routine newborn examination should also confirm that all the digits of both the hands and feet are present. Extra or missing fingers or toes should alert the examining doctor to look for other less obvious abnormalities. In addition, the opinion of a plastic surgeon should normally be obtained.

- **Club foot** – In this condition, the entire foot, including the heel, is twisted inwards. The most common cause of a club foot is pressure on the foot while the baby is squashed within the womb. In such a situation, it is possible to manipulate the foot back to the normal position. The parents will be taught what to do and within a few days the foot will be returned to the normal position without further problem. If gentle movement cannot restore the usual anatomy, the foot should be splinted back to the normal position, or occasionally surgery may be necessary. The management of this condition, like congenital dislocation of the hip, should be under the supervision of an orthopaedic surgeon.

- **Umbilical cord** – this life-sustaining structure nourishes the baby until birth. Then it becomes redundant as the baby assumes an independent existence. After the cord has been cut at birth, a stump about 2–4cm will be left. This will rapidly shrivel, dry up and will eventually turn black. It is important to keep the nappy below the level of the cord and not to cover it, to reduce the chances of an infection developing in the wound site. The stump should be cleaned daily either with water or an antiseptic. Soon the rest of the cord will just fall off, leaving the wound to heal and form the belly button.

HEEL PRICK TEST

At about the seventh day of life either the health visitor or the mid-wife will take a drop of blood from the baby's heel and place it on a card. This is sent to the lab for analysis and screening, usually for phenylketonuria (Guthrie test) and an under-active thyroid. In some areas cystic fibrosis is also routinely screened from the same sample.

Jaundice

In the first few days of life, the body can be temporarily over-whelmed by the sheer volume of products from blood metabolism. This leads to a transient accumulation of a compound called bilirubin and it is this substance that gives skin the distinct yellow discoloration.

The depth of colour is a rough indicator of the intensity of the jaundice but a more accurate picture can be arrived at by a blood test which measures the concentration of bilirubin in the blood. Treatment of babies with abnormally high levels often involves exposing them to a special type of light which converts the bilirubin to a non-toxic substance which is easily disposed of by the body. If jaundice were to persist for more than 14 days in a baby born at the correct date, doctors would also want to exclude the possibility of other serious illnesses which can cause jaundice, including various infections and liver abnormalities. If left untreated, severe jaundice can cause deafness, brain damage or may even prove to be fatal.

Skin rashes and birthmarks

- **Milia** are white pimples commonly found on the nose and cheeks. They are harmless and will clear up with no treatment.
- **Mongolian blue spots** are more common in children with dark skin. The name refers to pigmented areas, often at the base of the back or in the buttocks, and can resemble bruises. Again, they are harmless and will slowly fade during childhood.
- **Stork marks**, also called salmon patches, are commonly found around the eyes and the nape of the neck. Affected areas around the eyes usually disappear when the baby is about one year old, while those at the neck may persist, though some may fade with time.
- **Strawberry marks** can, as the name suggests, resemble a strawberry with a raised red appearance, speckled with small white areas. They can start from small spots at birth and grow rapidly. Most disappear by the age of seven years.
- **Port wine stains** are permanent irregular dark red patches. In contrast to strawberry marks, the skin is usually not raised. Treatment is best managed by camouflage and occasionally by laser.

Babies with medical problems

Most newborn babies have no problems, but a few babies are born with abnormalities and illnesses, sometimes revealed by antenatal screening. With most conditions the precise cause is not known but a hereditary influence or an environmental factor may be responsible: for instance, as a result of exposure to a substance or an infective agent during pregnancy. Of the various medical problems that can affect babies, some are relatively common while others are rare and beyond the scope of this book. The more frequently occurring conditions are looked at below.

Spina bifida and hydrocephalus

The likelihood of a child being born with spina bifida can be reduced by the mother taking folic acid (see page 11) before conception and during the earlier part of pregnancy. If the child does develop the condition, it is usually picked up during pregnancy by routine ultrasound scanning. Spina bifida is an abnormality in the rear part of the spine which causes part of the bony spinal column to be missing. There are a whole host of variations of this condition, from inconsequential irregularities to severe cases, where the spinal cord can be exposed. Depending on the damage to the spinal cord, paralysis below the level of the defect can occur. In addition, there can be interference to the flow of the spinal fluid which circulates around the brain and the spinal cord and this can lead to increased pressure in the brain – hydrocephalus. Surgery may be needed soon after birth to rectify the spinal defect and many different specialists may be involved, including an orthopaedic surgeon, a paediatric surgeon and a physiotherapist.

Hydrocephalus (which can be caused by conditions other than spina bifida) can be treated by placing a tube in the brain – a procedure often performed by a neurosurgeon – to drain off the excess fluid to another site in the body, sometimes the tummy.

Cleft lip and palate

The face is formed in the womb by separate areas growing and developing independently before meeting up with each other. In the case of a cleft lip and a cleft palate, the tissues that form the lip and the roof of the mouth – the palate – fail to unite.

A cleft lip is a split or a gap in the upper lip; it might be just a small notch or one which extends right up to the nostril. A cleft palate, slightly less common than a cleft lip, is a hole in the roof of the mouth and affects about 1 in 700 children. Some children have both a cleft lip and cleft palate.

Since so much of a child's beauty comes from its face, the sight of a cleft lip or a cleft palate can be devastating to the parents, so if your child is born with such a defect it is important that you are shown before-and-after pictures of treated children at an early stage to aleviate your worry. Fortunately, the outlook for children with such a disorder is good.

The first problem is one of establishing feeding, as the baby may have difficulty suckling. Special teats or a dental plate may help, and more than one method may need to be tried before the right one is found. Babies with this condition can feed successfully by breast and bottle.

The treatment is surgical and is often performed in stages, depending both on the surgeon and the degree of abnormality. In general, however, a cleft lip may be repaired when the baby is three months old and a cleft palate between about six and twelve months. Many children will require further facial surgery to the palate, lip or nose for cosmetic reasons or to facilitate speech. As the middle of the face grows dental treatment may be needed. Children with cleft palate are also at risk of glue ear – if left untreated this could adversely affect their hearing, so grommets are often inserted to treat the problem (see page 200).

There is more to treating a baby with a cleft palate than surgery alone. The surgeon is part of a team that will be involved as the years go by, including a dentist, a plastic surgeon and a speech therapist. Speech and language therapy can start at 18 months and speech will develop well in more than half of affected children. However, others experience difficulty with pronunciation: for instance, sounding p, b and t can be difficult. A hearing specialist may be brought in, too, as children with cleft palate are prone to hearing problems and ear infections.

Heart abnormalities

Heart disease is one of the most common abnormalities that a baby can be born with. The defect is sometimes picked up on a routine scan during pregnancy; in that case the unborn baby will be subjected to more detailed scans and if necessary will be delivered in a specialised unit.

Not every baby with a heart problem will need surgery and not every heart murmur is serious. A heart murmur is a vibration caused by an unusually turbulent blood flow and its presence alone does not necessarily mean the baby has a heart problem. If there is any doubt about how serious the murmur is, a chest x-ray and a heart tracing – an ECG and a ultrasound scan of the heart, similar to a pregnancy ultrasound scan – will be performed.

Many babies or children with heart murmurs will have no abnormality of the heart. Once it is established that a murmur is 'innocent' it can be safely ignored and the baby or child can be treated as normal with no limitations on his or her lifestyle.

Because of the complexity of the normal heart, there are numerous types of heart defect. The commoner ones include:

- a hole in the heart: this means the chambers of the heart have an abnormal communication. This may sometimes result in the blood not flowing through the lungs – if the lungs are bypassed the blood will be deficient in oxygen, giving rise to a 'blue baby'. There are a wide variety of holes in the heart, depending on their size and situation. Some will require surgical closure, while others will close spontaneously over a period of several years
- a narrowing of one of the four main heart valves guarding either an exit or entry to one of the heart chambers
- a narrowing of one of the main arteries leading from the heart
- a collection of multiple abnormalities – this tends to be more serious.

Sometimes a heart problem may not be picked up at the routine check straight after the baby is born, but a little later when he or she shows undue breathlessness, especially after feeding or crying, and having difficulty with finishing feeds and, as a result, failing to thrive. Excessive sweating can sometimes be a significant symptom of heart failure.

Waiting for your child to receive surgical treatment is naturally a worrying time. Many parents fear a sudden collapse if their child deteriorates. In practice, this is uncommon – a baby will usually show signs of a deterioration by slowing down generally and not thriving.

Cerebral palsy

Cerebral palsy is thought to affect about one baby in 500. It is a condition in which the brain has been damaged either at birth or at some point during development in the womb, resulting in problems with movement or posture. Some babies are only marginally affected while others are very disabled. The brain damage does not worsen as the baby gets older although the effects change as the child develops. A child may also have learning difficulties and problems with hearing or seeing and some may suffer from epilepsy. Much research remains to be done.

Treatment involves a wide range of health professionals: physiotherapists, occupational therapists, paediatricians, audiologists and speech therapists, to name but a few. Because of their disabilities some children may have special educational needs though this can be difficult to assess. Some severely physically disabled children may have normal intelligence masked by their handicaps.

First-year problems

Described below are the problems that all babies have before they are one year old, such as teething pain and nappy rash; also other conditions that only some babies will encounter.

Bowel problems

Just like adults, infants can have tummy problems but the causes are significantly different. An infant who is sick may simply have a problem with feeding and be swallowing excessive air. If not properly winded he may regurgitate his feeds. Larger feeds, more frequent feeds or a larger hole in the teat may be all that is required.

A not uncommon cause of vomiting is **reflux** of the stomach contents back into the gullet. This is caused by a faulty valve at the junction of the stomach and gullet, and usually settles by the age of one year without specific treatment.

Bowel obstruction in a baby is uncommon; it can be caused by loops of bowel being trapped inside a hernia or by a condition called intussusception, in which a loop of bowel folds inwards on itself, causing the baby to have screaming attacks and pass bloodstained mucus via the back passage. It is an easy diagnosis to miss but it can cause the baby or child to be very ill.

Gastro-enteritis is a relatively common condition which often causes sickness, diarrhoea and tummy pain. It is caused by an inflammation in the bowels commonly due to a virus or a bacteria.

The main danger is loss of fluids causing dehydration and an upset in the delicate balance of the body's minerals. Dehydration, especially in the early stages, is very difficult to detect in babies and young children.

In children under the age of two the detrimental effects of gastro-enteritis may not only be harder to detect but may be more severe. Again, it is always wise to seek medical advice sooner rather than later. In this age group, diarrhoea and vomiting persisting for more than a few hours should normally be assessed by a doctor. In an older child, parents can wait to observe the child a little longer.

If the child is still unwell after seeing the doctor, even if it was only relatively recently, and you are not sure what to do, seek advice again. For more about treating gastro-enteritis see page 195.

Infants and young children suffering a bout of gastro-enteritis need careful watching. It is a condition which although common should be given the utmost respect. Vomiting may be part of a seemingly unrelated problem such as an ear infection or a water-works infection, so if your baby keeps on vomiting seek your doctor's advice sooner rather than later.

Occasionally, as a result of the gastro-enteritis, a few infants and young children will suffer damage to the lining of the bowels. This will result in loose stools which could imply that the original tummy bug has not completely gone. In fact, what has happened is that certain sugars, particularly lactose which is found in milk, have not been absorbed and are acting like a laxative. This is usually short-lived. A lactose-free milk preparation may solve the problem but should be used only under medical supervision.

Breathing problems

Infection of the respiratory tract in the older infant is very common, with pre-school children having three to six or more **colds** a year. There is no specific treatment and antibiotics will not make any difference. Other babies and young children are often regularly catarrhal. Despite being a common problem the exact nature and of cause of catarrh is often unclear.

Almost all babies and children suffer from **coughs** at some point. Many doctors frown on cough medicines, doubting their effectiveness, and will not prescribe them; they are anyway limited to what cough preparations they can prescribe on the NHS. However, there is still a large market for cough medicines. Check with the pharmacist the suitability of any preparation you buy over the counter, particularly when dealing with young children and babies. A soothing hot drink with lemon and honey is tasty, inexpensive and a good way to make both parent and child feel that something is being done.

Tonsillitis and **sore throats** are relatively common. Drinks rich in vitamin C have been advocated as both a preventative measure and a treatment for colds, though this is still controversial.

Ear infections are another common cause of non-specific ill health though some babies and older children will be able localise the discomfort to the ear (see page 182).

Croup is characterised by spasms of barking cough, difficulty in breathing and noisy breathing called stridor, brought about by inflammation and partial obstruction of the voice box, airways in the neck and upper lungs. It is usually caused by a viral infection so antibiotics have very little effect. Some children may improve if they spend some time in a steamy bathroom. If the child is distressed or the breathing difficulties worsen, or if you are worried, seek medical advice.

Acute bronchiolitis

This is an infection which affects the small tubes deep within the lungs. The condition often occurs in epidemics during the winter time, commonly in babies under one. Initially, the baby may just have a cough but may then deteriorate, with laboured breathing coupled with obvious distress. Respiratory Syncytial Virus is the most common culprit. If the child is unwell he or she may need to be admitted to hospital.

Colic

A baby cries if he is hungry, cold or ill. Colic is a term used when a baby cries or screams, often uncontrollably, for no obvious reason. Typically, colic attacks occur, in both boys and girls, between the ages of three weeks and three to four months, most commonly in the evening. Sometimes the baby's knees are drawn up as if in pain.

The exact cause is unknown, but one theory is that patches of tissue in the baby's bowel – Peyer's patches – swell up in response to a changing diet, causing bowel spasms and pain. Too rapid feeding, overfeeding or insufficient winding are also thought to be possible causes.

Colic is a great source of parental anxiety. The temptation is to go to the crying baby and offer a feed, if only to get some peace during the early hours. You may get better results if you:

- massage the baby's stomach gently
- provide motion in the form of a rocking chair, a pram or a car ride
- hum, sing or play music
- give the baby some visual stimulation such as a mobile above the cot.

On the whole, drug treatment has little, if any, effect. Many remedies have been tried including dimethicone (Infacol), gripe-water and paracetamol elixir. Often the act of giving the baby something may be more helpful to the parent rather than to the baby.

The two important things to remember about colic are that it will resolve in time and that it will have no lasting harmful effects on the baby. If it is all getting too much for you, speak to your health visitor or your GP, or ask a friend or relative to take the baby for a while, just to give you a break.

One final word of warning: don't always assume that a screaming baby's distress is due to colic. Consider other possibilities and if necessary contact a doctor. Many other illnesses have initially been blamed on teething or colic until the true diagnosis has been discovered.

Failure to thrive

A baby is weighed at birth and at regular intervals thereafter. In the first few days there may be a temporary fall in weight as the baby adjusts to independent life. However, the birth weight is usually regained by the end of the first week and by six months the baby's birth weight may have doubled.

Changes in weight are recorded by the midwife or health visitor or at the child health clinic. It can be a source of great concern to parents if it is not satisfactory. There are many possible causes for poor weight gain or even weight loss in an infant. For more about failure to thrive, see also page 111.

Feeding

The baby may not be gaining weight because of inadequate feeding, inadequate winding, or regurgitation of feeds. There may be a problem such as a hiatus hernia: part of the baby's stomach slides up into the chest through the diaphragm, causing the stomach contents to be regurgitated. A change in the feeding regime or, if the baby is bottle-fed, the addition of thickening agents to the formula may help.

Some babies encounter feeding difficulties whether they are taking in breastmilk or formula milk. They may not absorb the nutrients for some reason and will therefore fail to thrive. For instance, babies and children with cystic fibrosis will fail to absorb vital components of the diet such as fat and vitamins. This malabsorption can be corrected but it is important that these children are identified.

Occasionally intolerance to proteins in cow's milk can occur, provoking sickness and diarrhoea, and resulting in failure to thrive; it can be corrected by prescribing alternative feeds.

Illness

Poor weight gain may simply be the consequence of an illness such as gastro-enteritis, or a urinary or respiratory infection. Once the infection has passed, the child will start to regain weight. Chronic conditions such as heart disease can also be associated with poor general health and poor weight gain.

Pyloric stenosis

One condition which can occur in the first four to six weeks of life is pyloric stenosis. In this condition, the outlet of the stomach – the pylorus, which is a circle of muscle – becomes swollen and blocks the passage of food from the stomach into the bowel. Symptoms of this are profuse 'projectile' vomiting which occurs soon after every feed. A baby vomiting in this way needs to be assessed by a doctor – if pyloric stenosis is diagnosed an operation will be necessary to relieve the obstruction. Though worrying for parents, it is not a major operation and the outcome is successful.

Serious conditions

Serious conditions such as heart disease and kidney disease are very rare. Modern antenatal screening detects most cases before birth enabling treatment to be planned for. Babies whose conditions are yet to be diagnosed will fail to gain weight adequately until the condition is recognised and dealt with.

Social factors

A physically healthy infant may be restless, irritable and a poor feeder if there is unhappiness around in the home. Unhappy relationships or the mother's post-natal depression may contribute to this. Support from the family, particularly grandparents, the health visitor and the doctor may all help to settle the problem. Occasionally, the baby and possibly the mother too will be admitted to hospital to give the mother a rest and some sleep. This can break the vicious circle of tired mother/irritable child.

Febrile convulsions

A febrile convulsion is a type of fit or seizure caused by a fever. In general terms, a fit is an electrical disturbance in the brain which can give rise to abnormal muscular activity. It can be caused by a sudden rise in temperature – it is thought that the brains of young children are more sensitive than older ones to such rises in temperature. The fever is often the result of a respiratory infection.

A typical attack will begin with a loss of consciousness. The first phase is called the tonic phase, in which the baby's body becomes stiff. This is followed by the clonic phase, in which there is a rhythmic jerking of the baby's body, particularly the arms and legs. During the fit, the baby may temporarily stop breathing, producing a blue tinge around the mouth known as cyanosis. After a few minutes, which may seem like hours, the fit is over. The baby may be drowsy for a period of time – this is known as the post-ictal phase.

Febrile convulsions are by far the most common cause of fits in children; 4 per cent of children have at least one febrile convulsion, and some may have recurrent attacks. The first febrile convulsion usually occurs in the first three years, with about 25 per cent of such convulsions occurring for the first time before the age of one year. There is often a family history of fits.

Benign febrile convulsions can recur so parents will be given advice on how to control fever in future illnesses. Even repeated febrile convulsions in childhood are usually not due to epilepsy and they are likely to stop by the age of five or six years. It is

FEBRILE CONVULSIONS – WHAT TO DO

As with most problems, prevention is often better than cure. If your baby is ill with a fever, take measures to reduce the temperature such as sponging him or her with tepid water, removing layers of clothing and giving a medicine such as paracetamol elixir. An unexplained fever which does not settle should prompt you to seek medical advice. However, fits can occur despite these measures.

A fit is a frightening experience and most parents will understandably reach for the phone and dial 999, particularly if this is the baby's first fit. By the time the ambulance arrives the fit is likely to have finished.

If a fit lasts less than 10 minutes and the baby recovers completely, the attack is regarded as benign and the main worries are over. However, your baby should still be taken to hospital where the cause of the fit will need to be ascertained and treated accordingly. Doctors will check for certain serious conditions such as meningitis or encephalitis.

After a benign fit has ceased, the baby's fever can be controlled by sponging with cool water and keeping clothing to a minimum. Your baby will be examined and various tests such as blood tests or a chest x-ray may be carried out. Your baby may need further treatment with paracetamol and possibly antibiotics.

If a fit continues for more than 15–20 minutes – by this time it is likely that help will have arrived or your baby will have reached hospital – steps must be taken to stop the fit, otherwise the baby's brain could be starved of vital oxygen. A sedative drug such as diazepam will be given, usually by injection into a vein, but if this is difficult a liquid form of the drug – rectal diazepam – will be inserted via the baby's bottom. This is absorbed into the bloodstream and carried to the brain, where it acts as a sedative and reduces the abnormal electrical impulses that are causing the fit. The baby's mouth will be inspected and any secretions will be gently cleared by a small plastic tube inserted in the baby's mouth. The baby will then be admitted to hospital, observed and given further drugs if necessary.

uncommon for a child suffering from febrile convulsions to go on to develop epilepsy in later life.

After a serious fit, or if fits are very frequent, doctors may advise that the baby or child is started on regular medication to prevent fits, at least until later in childhood. These medicines are known as anti-convulsants and are taken daily. They are carefully monitored, often with blood tests to measure the level in the bloodstream, so that the right amount is delivered.

Hearing and vision

When a baby is born the two critical senses of hearing and vision are not fully developed but take time to mature. Newborn babies startle but are unable to localise the source of the sound; that happens at around 4–6 months. They soon start to recognise their carer's voice and by seven months they should be able to discriminate between different sounds. This normal development is essential for the acquisition of language, so it is essential to detect a deaf baby as soon as possible. If you are in any doubt that your baby cannot hear, seek early advice from your GP or health visitor and do not wait for the routine hearing test that is usually performed by the health visitor at about seven months. Many experienced doctors take the view that if parents suspect that their baby cannot hear, then more often than not they are right.

Sophisticated tests can establish if the baby cannot hear and babies or children with impaired hearing are often prescribed a hearing aid to maximise whatever hearing they have.

Vision is rather crudely developed at birth although babies are able to screw up their eyes if they are exposed to sudden bright. They have some colour perception but this is not fully developed until they are about three months old. Many people assume that newborn babies cannot see – in fact, they have limited vision but they cannot focus for different distances. As the visual processing centre of the brain develops, babies start to understand more about their environment and by about one year they have pretty good vision. In the first few weeks a baby begins to see images and fixes on them. The baby will usually recognise his or her mother's face first and will respond by smiling.

Just as with hearing, it is important to identify babies with any form of visual impairment. Sometimes there may be a family history of eye disease or other abnormalities which will alert doctors to look specifically for visual problems. Some babies may show subtle signs of visual impairment: for example, the baby may startle when touched because he could not see the person approaching, or the baby's eyes may roll excessively.

Any doubt about vision, no matter how unsure the parents are, must be taken seriously. This means a medical assessment, often by specialists.

Squint

Normally, both eyes look in the same direction at one time and the images formed by both eyes are used equally by the brain in order to see. The eyes are moved by a series of muscles around the eye. These ocular muscles usually work together and with equal strength.

A squint (strabismus) occurs when, for a variety of reasons, the two eyes are not aligned and not working together. Excessive action of the muscles can pull the eye inwards – a convergent squint – or outwards – a divergent squint.

If you want to check whether your baby has a squint, with your baby awake and quiet, look at the eyes. Notice where light reflections appear on the eyes in relation to the pupil (the circular opening in the middle of the eye which can vary in size to allow the correct amount of light to enter the eye). Normally the light reflects at the same position on both eyes, but with a squint the light reflex will appear offset on one eye.

In some babies, the inner part of the skin of the upper eyelid next to the nose is prominent and gives the appearance of a squint which is not actually there at all. The light reflex test will clear up any confusion. Your doctor or health visitor will check the baby's eyes at the six-week check and subsequent routine checks.

If a squint is detected your doctor will refer your baby to an ophthalmologist. He or she will confirm the diagnosis and exclude other rare conditions such as brain disorders and cataracts.

The brain suppresses the visual information from the squinting eye so as to avoid double vision. It is important to treat the squint quickly – otherwise the eye will be irrevocably suppressed. The weak eye is said to be amblyopic.

There are four main treatments:

- **Correction of optical problems** – a squint may simply be due to longsightedness, for instance. The use of corrective spectacles may be all that is necessary. As the vision in the weak eye is improved the brain will use both eyes equally and vision will develop normally.
- **Occlusion of the good eye** – patching of the good eye may be

necessary if spectacles alone are not sufficient to correct the squint. This improves the function of the 'lazy' eye.

- **Eye muscle exercises** – these can be used to prevent the eye muscles from getting into the habit of making incorrect movements which accentuate the squint.
- **Surgery** – if the other measures fail a small operation may be necessary either to strengthen a weak eye muscle or to weaken an overactive one.

Nappy rash

Most babies suffer from nappy rash at some time. Often it is mild, but in some babies it can be severe and repeated. It is not always due to poor care and can be very difficult to avoid. Despite this, many parents feel defensive when their child has a nappy rash, thinking it implies that they have not taken proper care of the baby, but that is far from the case – even the most meticulous of parents will see nappy rash on their child. If nappy rash is due to neglect there are usually other signs of poor care or abuse.

Nappy rash can be regarded as an acceptable complication of wearing nappies. It can be due to one of three main causes, or a mixture of two or even all three.

- Pure napkin dermatitis, as it is formally called, is due to the irritant effect of a wet nappy against the skin. Germs which are normally present in the bowel motions react with urine to produce ammonia which is alkaline, irritant and produces a characteristic smell. The angry-looking red rash affects the skin of the nappy area that is in contact with the dirty nappy but does not extend into the skin creases in that area.
- Candidiasis, commonly known as thrush, is a fungal infection which attacks the already inflamed skin surface, causing an additional infection. With this type of infection, the rash does extend into the skin creases and may also have smaller spots away from the main rash, called satellite spots.
- Finally, a rash in the nappy area may be due to irritation or infection of a skin condition which is already present, such as eczema.

Prevention of nappy rash is important. Frequent nappy changes to keep the area clean and dry for as long as possible will help. If possible, leave the baby with no nappy at all for some of the time. To prevent accidents, lay the baby on a towel or changing mat. For an older infant who is crawling or walking, choose a time just after you have had to change the nappy anyway, and be prepared for accidents.

If your baby is in terries, place a one-way nappy liner next to the skin and wash the nappies in a non-biological detergent. Clean the baby's bottom with cotton wool and water rather than soap or baby wipes, and avoid applying any extra irritants: talc or baby powder is not really necessary.

After cleaning, apply a simple protective cream such as zinc and castor oil cream. You may have to experiment with different creams – ask a pharmacist – to find the one that suits your baby best. The cream should be lightly applied, as too much cream can clog up the nappy or the liner, stopping it from absorbing moisture effectively.

If the rash shows no signs of improvement, if the skin creases are affected, or if there is blistering, seek the advice of your doctor. It may be that your baby needs a more sophisticated type of treatment. Many different creams and ointments are available, many of them steroid-based. If used according to instructions and as a short-term measure they are entirely safe.

Sticky eyes (conjunctivitis)

This is a common problem in infants and although it may look unsightly it is not usually serious, and the baby is not usually ill. For more information, see page 165.

Teething

The first set of teeth, the milk teeth, forms within the gums before birth. Often babies cut their first tooth, commonly one of the middle upper or lower teeth, at about six months, though this can vary. See also Chapter 7.

Babies become disturbed in a variety of ways when their teeth start to erupt through the gums. There is disagreement between some doctors and parents what symptoms can and cannot be attributed to teething. Teething may stimulate drooling and will affect some babies more than others. If a baby is a big drooler, rashes may develop because of the irritation of the saliva on the skin. To reduce the chances of this occurring, regularly clean the chin with a towel or a bib. If a patch of skin is dry and irritated, use some simple barrier cream, and if that fails have a word with your doctor or pharmacist.

Some babies will bite when they are teething, preferring a hard object such as a finger or a teething ring. This brings relief to both the baby and the concerned parent. Other babies may respond by reducing their feeding, but if the lack of appetite persists for more than a few days don't always assume that this is due to teething and seek medical advice.

Symptoms like diarrhoea, nappy rash and a fever have all been attributed to teething. Some doctors do not accept this while many mothers are convinced that these symptoms have a definite connection with their baby's teething. If your baby has a fever or diarrhoea keep an open mind as to whether it is due to teething or to another illness altogether. Treat each symptom on its own merit.

There are more treatments for teething than for almost any other condition but here are a few common ones. Many babies like to bite on something and obtain relief from the pressure on the gums. A plastic (not wooden) railing of a cot, an adult finger, a toy or food may soothe the baby. Always supervise the baby when using an object like a toy or food and make sure the baby is in a sitting position while chewing. Sometimes junior paracetamol may give relief where nothing else works. This can be particularly useful in the middle of the night when the parents are desperate for some sleep. Avoid rubbing any medication on the baby's gums unless it has been recommended by a pharmacist or a doctor.

Aromatherapy has been advocated as a treatment for teething. Adding one or two drops of lavender oil to a vaporiser in the baby's nursery may help. Some homeopathic powders have also been advocated.

Undescended testicle

As a baby boy develops in his mother's womb, his testicles begin to grow inside his tummy, close to the kidneys. As the pregnancy progresses, the testicles gradually descend towards their intended place in the sac (scrotum). At birth the testicles will have descended correctly into the scrotum in all but 10 per cent of boys. In this group the testicles of most will descend within the first few weeks of life, but about 2 per cent of boys at the age of one year will still have an absent or undescended testicle.

It is quick and easy for parents to examine the testicles in their new baby boy. This is best done in a warm environment during a nappy change or while the baby is being bathed. Make sure your hands are warm and that the baby is relaxed.

The testicles will also be examined by the midwife, the health visitor or the doctor at the birth check and at any routine medical checks at the child health clinic. If you have any concerns, do not wait for the next routine medical check, but contact your health visitor or doctor for advice. If one or both testicles cannot be found in the scrotum then there are two possible explanations.

- **Retractile testicle** – the testicles can be pulled up into the groin by a reflex action in response to stimulation such as touch or exposure to cold. This is quite normal and with warmth and gentle massage, the testicle can be coaxed back down into the scrotum.
- **Undescended testicle** – a testicle that has not fully descended during development is commonly found in the groin but may still be inside the tummy. There is often a hernia present in these cases. If the testicle has descended far enough but in the wrong place it is described as 'maldescended'. In this situation it can be found in places such as the thigh or even in the other side of the scrotum.

Testicles needs to be maintained at a cooler temperature than the normal body temperature in order to mature properly. An undescended testicle, being within the body, is subjected to a higher temperature, which can have two possible adverse effects if the problem is not corrected.

First, the sperm-producing cells will not develop properly and future fertility may be impaired. Fertility will therefore depend on the other, normally sited, testicle's ability to produce sperm. An undescended testicle also has a higher risk – perhaps 40 times higher – of becoming cancerous in later life.

If your baby's testicle has not descended by 12 months, your doctor will refer him to a paediatric surgeon. If the testicle is undescended as opposed to retractile, the only real option is surgery. Once it has been located, whether by simple examination or a scan, an operation would be carried out. Opinions vary about the age at which surgery should be carried out. The age of five was the standard until recently but surgery is now being considered for boys of around two years old. Surgery is best left until the child is out of nappies to prevent complications such as irritation or infection of the wounds.

Orchidopexy

This is the commonest operation. The surgeon will attempt to bring the testicle down into its normal position so that it is fixed within the scrotum. This is a minor operation and can be done without the need for overnight admission.

Orchidectomy

Rarely, it is not possible to bring the testicle down into the scrotum in that manner. If the other testicle is normal and the undescended testicle is abnormal and poorly formed, complete removal of the testicle may be necessary.

Cot death

Cot death is also known as Sudden Infant Death Syndrome (SIDS).

In two-thirds of cases where a baby dies the cause can be ascertained. Babies most at risk are those born with inherited illnesses or birth defects, those with very low birth weight and very premature babies, and those with severe infections such as meningitis.

The remaining third of babies who die, however, do so without any warning. There is little or no sign of illness before death and at post-mortem examination no indication of any illness or abnormality which could have been responsible. These are the so-called cot-death babies.

The cause (or causes) of cot death remains unknown. Theories about respiratory infections or milk regurgitation have been put forward but never proven. Cot death usually occurs at home and during sleep, between the ages of one and twelve months. But cot deaths are rare: in England and Wales in 1993 there were 458 cases of unexplained death in infants under the age of one year. This number is smaller than that for deaths due to conditions such as meningitis, cystic fibrosis or leukaemia.

Recent research, both in the UK and elsewhere, such as Australia, New Zealand and Germany, has shown the following factors to be associated with a higher incidence of cot death:

- poor antenatal attendance and care
- mother smoking or taking illicit drugs during pregnancy
- prematurity
- smoking in the baby's home
- poor social circumstances
- bed-sharing with parent or parents
- overheating due to excessive bedding or clothing
- sleeping on the tummy
- urban areas
- winter months.

It was once thought that chemicals added as fire retardants to cot mattresses led to the production of toxic gases, increasing the risk of cot death. Recent research by several independent studies, however, has not been able to corroborate the original findings. The advice now is to use a firm mattress, kept clean and well aired.

In 1991 a national campaign was launched to increase awareness of the problem and provide advice for parents. The 'Back to sleep' campaign led to a two-thirds reduction in cot deaths between 1989 and 1993 in the UK. In the 1980s the rate of cot death was 2 cases per 1,000 live births. This has now dropped to 0.6 per 1,000 live births. Those parents whose baby may be at a higher risk of cot death can be identified and given extra support and advice from midwives, health visitors and doctors during and after pregnancy.

THE CURRENT ADVICE FOR REDUCING THE RISK OF COT DEATHS:

- place babies on their back or side to sleep
- avoid overheating the baby
- avoid smoky environments
- contact a doctor if the baby is unwell.

Help and advice is available from the Foundation for the Study of Infant Deaths*; there is also a 24-hour cot death helpline* for both families and professionals.

CHAPTER 3

GETTING YOUR CHILD IMMUNISED

SOON after having a baby, when the experiences of giving birth and all the associated emotions are so fresh in the mind, the mother is suddenly under pressure to start making decisions about immunisation. All parents naturally want the best for their child and are worried about putting their baby at risk.

What is immunisation?

To all intents and purposes, the words immunisation and vaccination mean the same thing. Immunisation may be active or passive. Passive immunisation takes place when antibodies – protective chemicals produced by the body's immune system – from another source are given to the patient, to produce short-term protection against a specific illness (e.g. to protect you on holiday against hepatitis).

Active immunisation involves a much more sophisticated process. Most germs are chemically quite complicated and on their surfaces have compounds which the body's immune system recognises as foreign. This provokes the body's immune system into producing antibodies and other chemical defences to repel the invader.

It is possible in the laboratory to modify these bugs so that they still have the chemicals that promote an immune response but are devoid of the toxic parts which make a person ill. The defensive substances produced by the body will react to either or both the neutered and virulent forms of the bug and so immunity is achieved. Vaccines are therefore collections of modified micro-organisms derived from the more virulent strains.

Most immunisations are given by injection, although poliomyelitis vaccine is given as drops into the mouth. The injection is usually delivered into the upper arm or the upper thigh.

The immunisation debate

Doctors are frequently asked if it is worthwhile to vaccinate when some of the immunisations themselves carry risks. The answer is yes: provided that certain precautions are taken the risks are very small indeed compared to the benefits. Side effects are rare but worth mentioning to put the risks into perspective.

These are some of the common concerns raised by parents uncertain as to whether to give their consent to vaccinations for their children. Always discuss any doubts with your health visitor or GP or clinic doctor.

Q *What about the danger of anaphylaxis?*

A Anaphylaxis is a severe reaction to foreign proteins found in vaccines as well as certain other substances, such as an insect bite or a peanut. In other words, it is an extreme form of allergy. Anaphylaxis can cause collapse, difficulty in breathing with low blood pressure and may require full resuscitation by a medical team or paramedics responding to a 999 call. It is important to differentiate an anaphylactic reaction from a simple faint, where the person concerned should make a spontaneous recovery.

In the case of immunisation, anaphylaxis can follow (very rarely) without warning from the injection within a matter of minutes and the person can become very ill. It is impossible to predict who will develop these reactions. However, it is important to put the problem into perspective: from 1992 to 1995, 87 cases of such a reaction were reported in the UK; this was out of 55 million vaccine doses supplied to health authorities. No fatalities were recorded.

Q *Is my child at risk of having a fever fit?*

A Despite some scare stories in the popular press, the fact is that very few children are at special risk of febrile convulsions (fever fits) from modern immunisation courses. Usually, the only precaution necessary is in cases where there is a history of such con-vulsions. Even then, all that is required is to make sure that for 24 hours after the immunisation the child is kept cool and is given paracetamol and sponged down if his or her temperature rises. (In the case of MMR vaccination, care should also be taken five to eleven days after administration – see below.) It is unnec-essary to decline immunisation because of a family history of allergy or fits.

Q *Is there a risk of brain damage?*

A Modern vaccines are extremely safe and are constantly being improved, so the risk is tiny.

Q *Wouldn't it be better if my child caught the disease naturally?*

A Before immunisation became commonplace, children picked up infectious diseases relatively young from other children. It is therefore important to remember that because these diseases are quite rare in immunised communities, the chances of children acquiring immunity by contact with other infected children are much reduced. Without a background immunity, an unimmunised adult who becomes infected is more likely to have a more severe form of the illness.

Q *Surely measles and German measles are harmless anyway?*

A This is a misconception. Measles can cause encephalitis, an inflammation of the brain. This can cause brain damage and may prove fatal. It is true that German measles (rubella) is a short-lived, mild infection in normal children but if a pregnant woman catches it, the effects on her unborn child are severe.

Q *Why can't I just immunise my child by introducing him or her to an infected person?*

A This is suitable for chickenpox; it can also be used for German measles, which is not likely to cause a serious illness in a small child. It is, however, a very uncertain method, with only a small success rate in developing antibodies, and it will mean that the child has to suffer the illness which may last for several days.

The rubella immunisation is much more successful in developing immunity, and is unlikely to cause much discomfort.

Q Were *the diseases that the vaccination programme is trying to eradicate not declining anyway?*

A Yes, but only because the number of immunised children is rising. If the immunisation rates were to drop the diseases would become prevalent again.

Q *Why do children have to be vaccinated so young when their immune systems are still developing?*

A Children are vaccinated at a young age precisely because the response to vaccination is most successful then.

Q *Can certain herbal treatments can be used as an alternative to vaccination?*

A There is no scientific evidence to support herbal or other alternatives to conventional immunisation and they are not recommended.

Q *What about children with compromised immune systems?*

A Some children may be given protection against illnesses that represent a specific danger to them because their defence systems may already be compromised by other illnesses. A good example is the use of pneumococcal immunisation in children who may not have a functioning spleen, perhaps because it has been removed through illness or injury; sometimes the spleen can be rendered non-functional by the presence of other diseases. Without the contribution of the spleen in fighting infection, these children are at a greater risk of an overwhelming infection.

Q *Are there other forms of immunisation?*

A Immunisations are also used when a child is at special risk. This could be when travelling abroad (for example, yellow fever), or when there is a risk that a specific illness may have been contracted (for example, giving rabies vaccine if a child may have been bitten abroad and there is a risk that the animal may have rabies).

Immunisation in the UK

Different countries have developed different immunisation programmes tailored to the needs of their individual communities. Even in the United Kingdom, until quite recently, different health authorities advised general practitioners and local authority clinics to use slightly varying regimes. However, there is now uniformity of advice across the country.

Until quite recently the only protection available was against polio, diphtheria, tetanus and whooping cough. Older children were offered protection against tuberculosis. Over the last few years this list has been expanded to include measles, mumps and rubella (German measles), which are usually given together in the one vaccine – MMR – and Hib (*Haemophilus influenzae* type b), a potential cause of meningitis, epiglottitis and septicaemia, which was introduced as recently as the early 1990s.

Immunisation schedule

You should receive a letter from your health visitor, GP or clinic to invite you to bring your child for each set of immunisations.

- **Diphtheria, tetanus, pertussis (DTP, combined vaccine), Hib and poliomyelitis**: the primary course consists of three doses – one each at two, three and four months of age
- **Measles, mumps, rubella (MMR, combined vaccine)**: can be given from 12 months of age onwards, usually between 12 and 15 months
- **Booster diphtheria and tetanus (combined vaccine) and polio; also MMR (second dose)**: given three years after the completion of the primary course, at between 3 and 5 years of age
- **BCG**: given as protection against tuberculosis between 10 and 14 years, although some children are offered the vaccination earlier if they are at particular risk; some health authorities give it routinely in infancy. (Before giving the BCG vaccine, a test for immunity is carried out – this is called the HEAF test. It consists of a mini-puncture of the skin in the forearm and shows whether or not the child has already got immunity to tuberculosis.)
- **Booster diphtheria and polio**: given between 13 and 18 years.

A detailed look at the immunisations

All diseases are undesirable, but there are particular reasons why we take precautions against some and not others. Immunisation is used where the threat of the illness is greater than the threat from the immunisation procedure and where an effective, safe and proven immunisation is available.

There are still many life-threatening conditions for which an immunisation programme would be desirable but either no specific immunisation exists or the one that is available is too risky to use.

Immunising your child brings benefits not only to your family but also to the community in which you live. The risks are small, and the benefits are tremendous.

The diseases for which a safe and effective prevention is available are as follows.

Diphtheria

Diphtheria is an infectious disease affecting mainly the throat and skin. The danger that it presents is that it can cause the formation of a membrane in the throat that may obstruct the airways, possibly fatally. It also releases toxins into the bloodstream which can affect the heart muscles as well as nervous tissue.

The number of cases in the UK has dropped dramatically since immunisation began. In 1940, 46,000 cases were reported, with 2,480 deaths. Between 1986 and 1995 only 38 cases were found, and there were no fatalities. Unfortunately, it is still common in some developing countries, while in some parts of the former Soviet Union the disease is re-emerging as a major problem. The increase in global travel has made immunisation against diptheria as necessary as it ever was. See also pages 178–80.

Vaccine risk
Swelling and redness at the site of the injection, tiredness and a transient fever are common, short-lived and harmless. Very rarely allergic reactions may occur.

Tetanus

Tetanus is an acute disease causing severe muscular rigidity and agonising contractions. It is often fatal despite the best medical care. Tetanus cannot be spread from person to person.

The spores of tetanus are present in the soil and can easily be transferred into the human body by often trivial injuries to the skin as well as via major trauma or burns. The tetanus bug likes airless sites, and wounds are ideal for its growth. It is impossible to eradicate the spores from the soil, and the only effective action is prevention by immunisation.

Vaccine risk
Swelling and redness at the site of the injection are common, short-lived and harmless. General reactions including lethargy, headache or muscle aches are rare and usually last only a short while. Very rarely allergic reactions may occur.

Pertussis

Pertussis is more widely known as whooping cough because it is characterised by spells of coughing spasms, often protracted, followed by a very typical whooping noise as the sufferer takes a deep breath. The danger is that it can cause severe pneumonia and vomiting which may dehydrate a small child or infant; on occasion it leads to brain damage. Most deaths occur in infants, but even in older or debilitated children it is a very dangerous illness. Pertussis is highly infectious. See also pages 248–50.

Whooping cough vaccine is the one most parents worry about, but the vaccines available are both safe (see 'Vaccine risk', below) and effective. In 1975, when vaccination rates of infants were about 30 per cent, over 100,000 cases of the illness occurred in England and Wales. By 1995, when vaccination rates had risen to 94 per cent in children under two years old, notifications of the disease had dropped to 1,873.

Vaccine risk
Swelling and redness at the site of the injection, malaise and a transient fever are common, short-lived and harmless.

More serious reactions including fits, brain damage and – very rarely – death have been reported after pertussis vaccine. However, analysis both in the USA and in the UK has shown that the numbers of cases related to recent immunisation are few and could just as easily have occurred by chance. The National Childhood Encephalopathy Study showed that in the United Kingdom between 1976 and 1979 a total of 1,182 children with a serious neurological illness were reported. Of this total only 39 children had been recently immunised against pertussis. That was no higher an incidence among the immunised children than among those who had not been recently immunised. It is also worth noting that complications like brain damage are considerably more common after having the disease itself than after immunisation.

Poliomyelitis

Poliomyelitis (polio) is one of a very small group of illnesses for which it is possible to provide immunity by giving the immunisation by mouth as opposed to by injection. Some people therefore assume that it is a less important or less dangerous disease. It is not.

Polio is an acute illness caused by a virus. It attacks nervous tissue and tends to multiply in the motor nerves (those that cause the muscles to contract) and can cause permanent paralysis of the affected muscles. It can also cause paralysis of some of the muscles used for breathing which if untreated may be fatal.

The vaccine given nowadays is a modified form of the live virus, and it is extremely safe and effective. In 1955, there were about 4,000 cases of paralytic poliomyelitis in England and Wales, whereas from 1985 to 1995 there were only 28 cases. The uptake for poliomyelitis vaccine in 1996 was 96 per cent of all children under the age of two.

Vaccine risk

Very rarely poliomyelitis (one in two million) has occurred in those who have received polio vaccine and those who were in very close contact with them. This could virtually be eliminated by making sure that close contacts of children being immunised, such as parents, grandparents and carers are themselves given oral poliomyelitis vaccine if they are not up-to-date on their polio vaccine.

Haemophilus influenzae type b

Despite its name, *haemophilus influenzae* type b (Hib) is nothing to do with 'flu. It is an important cause of meningitis. It can also cause septicaemia (infection of the blood), bone infections (osteomyelitis), pneumonia and heart problems.

49

Before immunisation was introduced, the incidence of the disease in children under five years old was one in six hundred. By 1995 there was a decline in infections of 96 per cent, and only one fatality. By 1996 it was estimated that 96 per cent of all children under two were immunised.

Vaccine risk
Swelling and redness at the site of the injection is common, short-lived and harmless.

Measles

Measles is a highly infectious acute viral illness. It may prove to be a relatively innocuous illness in some children, but there are serious and potentially fatal complications in a significant number of those infected. One in 5,000 children with measles may get encephalitis – inflammation of the brain – and this will prove fatal in one in six of those who do. Of those children who survive the encephalitis, nearly 40 per cent may be left with some form of brain damage.

Before immunisation was available, up to 800,000 cases were notified each year in England and Wales. By 1993, notifications had fallen to 9,612. Despite the possibility of a link to an increase in incidence of Crohn's Disease, the overwhelming evidence has not supported this and parents are well advised to continue with the MMR schedule. See also pages 216–19.

Vaccine risk
As for rubella – see below.

Mumps

Mumps is also an acute, infectious viral illness causing pain and swelling of either one or both parotid glands, which are located under the jaw line on both sides of the face and secrete saliva into the mouth . The complications of mumps are inflammation of the pancreas (a gland in the tummy), and inflammation of the ovaries in women and of the testicles in men. It can also cause meningitis or encephalitis. There is a strong suggestion that adult men contracting mumps can become sterile as a result of damage to the testicles. Mumps can also cause deafness at any age. See also page 223.

Vaccine risk
As for rubella – see below.

Rubella

Despite its alternative name, German measles, rubella is not related in any way to measles. Rubella is a mild infectious disease, which – before immunisation became common – was widespread among children in the 6-9-year-old age group.

The illness presents no danger to the child; but if a pregnant woman contracts rubella in the first eight to ten weeks of pregnancy, there is a 90 per cent chance of damage to the baby. Even up to 16 weeks of pregnancy there is a risk to the unborn child, albeit reduced. The possible effects on the developing baby are mental handicap, cataract, deafness, heart abnormalities, and damage to the brain, liver, lungs and bone marrow. This is a disaster which is absolutely avoidable by making sure that all women of childbearing age are immunised well before they become pregnant, and by reducing the pool of infection in the community by immunising all children.

Vaccine risk
The combined measles, mumps and rubella vaccine is known as MMR. Following the first dose of MMR, fever and/or a rash may occur, usually about a week after immunisation, which will last for a few days at most. In rare instances febrile convulsions (fever fits) occur six to eleven days after the MMR was given. This is thought to be due to the measles component, as the pattern is identical to that occurring when measles vaccine is given alone. It is worth watching for a fever from day five to day eleven, and giving paracetamol liquid at the first sign of a temperature.

Reactions to the second MMR injection are far fewer, but the same precautions as for the first injection should be taken.

Tuberculosis

Human tuberculosis may affect any part of the body, but 75 per cent of cases involve primarily the lungs. In the UK it is spread mainly by breathing in infected particles from the breath of those with the disease. It usually requires prolonged contact with the infected source, but not necessarily. Effective treatment exists for most people who have the illness, and deaths from tuberculosis have declined dramatically owing to the immunisation programme. It is still, however, a very dangerous disease.

Vaccine risk

The Bacillus Calmette-Guérin (BCG) vaccine against tuberculosis is usually given to schoolchildren at around 13 years of age, in schools or at special centres throughout the UK by trained doctors, but it is given earlier if a child is at special risk: for example, if any close family members have tuberculosis.

BCG is a tried and trusted vaccine and reactions to it are extremely rare.

Holiday jabs

If you are taking your child abroad seek advice from your GP or practice nurse in good time concerning requirements for immunisations.

CHAPTER 4

YOUR CHILD'S HEALTH AND DEVELOPMENT

THE GROWTH and development of every child in Britain is monitored under the Child Health Surveillance Programme. This is primarily a preventative programme focusing on healthy babies and children, flagging up when they are due for immunisation and recording their progress; it involves parents and many members of the health team. It is not a service for children who are ill – they should be seen by their GP in the normal way.

Information about health checks and immunisations is gathered on a large computer system. A broad team of specialists in dentistry, speech, hearing and vision are also linked into the programme. Each child is allocated to a designated professional who will carry out the developmental assessments. This may be the community health doctor, the GP, the health visitor (for under-fives) or the school nurse (for over-fives). In each case the health professional should contact the family to make appointments. The precise arrangements may vary from area to area.

Nowadays, many GPs run child health surveillance clinics and increasingly they have become the main providers of this programme. However, you have the choice of attending a community-based clinic instead – these are headed by community health doctors. Convenience of location and opening times may be your deciding factor. One main advantage of seeing your GP is that you know the staff and are familiar with the surroundings. Many GP-based clinics are run in conjunction with the health visitor.

The little red book

Since the early 1990s, most areas have been using this book, the parent-held child health record, in which to record details of each child's health. It is handed over to the mother soon after the baby is born. Keep it with you, perhaps in the baby's changing bag, as it contains important information. As your child gets older it can just be taken to health appointments.

Any health professional who sees your child should write in the little red book. There are specific places for immunisations and developmental and growth assessments to be recorded. If your child sees a doctor or specialist who does not write in the book you can jot down anything important, such as the date of starting a course of antibiotics.

The health visitor

Every family with a child under five years has automatic access to a named health visitor, who is a key member of the Child Health Surveillance Programme. Health visitors are employed by the health authority or NHS trust and then allocated to a GP practice, a hospital or a geographical area.

Qualified nurses with extra training, health visitors are different from most nurses in that they see people when they are well and help keep them well. They are available for advice and support about anything to do with family health. Most of their work focuses on the health and development of children under five years though they may continue to see families with children over five who have special needs (see page 69). In hospitals it is the liaison health visitors who offer this service as well as passing on information to the named health visitors about admissions to Accident and Emergency and the wards.

When do I see the health visitor?

- In pregnancy, at either the surgery or parentcraft classes, or she may contact you.
- Every family is offered a home visit 10–14 days after a baby is born.
- After this the frequency of visits depends on the health visitor, the family and the local policy.

- It may be left up to you to contact your health visitor if you would like advice or support.
- Health visitors run drop-in clinics, or you can phone their office for an appointment.
- In most areas a health visitor will contact you to carry out routine developmental and growth assessments of your child. Some of these reviews are shared with the GP – which ones depends on your local area policy.
- If you register a child under five years with a new GP you should automatically be contacted by your new health visitor.
- The health visiting service is *offered* to families with children under five years. You can decide not to have any contact with a health visitor, but if you do so the GP and health visitor's manager have to be notified.

What will the health visitor want to know about us?
The health visitor will probably want to know some basic information about your family, for example names and ages of family members, history of illnesses or conditions affecting health, housing situation, employment situation, family support. This helps her get to know you as a family and see how best she can be of service to you.

Do health visitors come to check that we are suitable parents?
Health visitors are not there to judge you but to help you make informed choices about your family's health. Like all professionals working with children, they have a duty to try to protect children from significant harm, so if they have reason to believe that a child is in danger they must share the information with social services. Before doing so, the health visitor would try to discuss her concerns with the child's parent or parents. Health visitors are very aware of the ups and downs of family life and do not expect families to live in perfect harmony.

What can I ask the health visitor?
Basically, anything that you are not sure about, however small. Here are some common topics:

- **Child health** – growth, speech, hearing, vision, crawling/walking, feeding problems with either breast or formula milk, sleep-

ing, weaning, reducing the risk of cot death, immunisations, safety and accident prevention, playgroups and nurseries, nappy rash, play, teething, toilet training, physical appearance, constipation, diarrhoea, temper tantrums, behavioural problems.
- **Family health** – sibling rivalry, diet, exercise, postnatal depression, contraception, sexual health, reducing risks of heart disease, HIV prevention, cancer screening, where to get advice on housing or benefits, local groups. Health visitors tend to have good information about services in their area and if they cannot help you directly they will usually know the best person for you to contact.

What happens when my child reaches five?

The responsibility for monitoring your child's health passes to the **school nurse** when your child reaches the age of five, but it is likely that by this stage any problem will have been identified and passed on to the school team anyway. In many areas children now see the school doctor only if they have an identified problem, and their hearing and eye tests will be performed by the school nurse. For this reason it is important to let the school nurse or your GP know if you have any concerns about your child's health.

School nurses are all trained nurses, some of whom have completed specific extra training geared to school nursing. They are involved with health education, covering smoking, sex education and HIV prevention, but can also advise on individual problems such as bedwetting or difficult behaviour. You can contact your child's school nurse via the school itself or through your local community health service.

Growth and development

A healthy child should grow, increasing in both weight and size, right from birth through to adulthood. The rate of growth will naturally fluctuate: it can be interrupted by physical illness, an inadequate diet, psychological trauma and specific growth disorders.

An average growth pattern
- During the first six months a baby grows rapidly, on average more than doubling his or her birth weight.

- This slows over the next six months so that on average at one year a baby is three times his or her birth weight.
- The growth in the first year is not always steady but may happen in spurts; for instance, a baby may wake in the night for an extra feed for a week and then return to the previous pattern, so will put on more weight during that short period.
- Over the second year weight gain is much slower but height increases. This explains the very obvious change in shape and proportion between a baby and a toddler.
- Between two years and puberty the rate of growth is relatively slower and steadier although growth spurts may still be evident; a child may suddenly grow out of all his clothes or jump quickly on to the next shoe size.
- The rate of growth increases at puberty to coincide with many changes in the female and male bodies. These changes can be alarming for both the child and the parents, particularly if puberty begins – as is becoming more and more common – before the age of 11.

Why is measurement of growth important?

Measurement of growth is used as an indicator of the state of a child's health but is really useful only when viewed in conjunction with other aspects of the child's behaviour and situation. Problems with growth will rarely be the only sign of ill health but may confirm that another symptom – diarrhoea, for example – needs further investigation. Once a problem of ill health has been diagnosed, measurement of growth – such as regular weight checks – is an important confirmation that treatment is working.

How is growth measured?

Three measurements are used routinely to determine satisfactory growth in children.

- **Weight** can fluctuate as a result of many factors and in itself is not a reliable indicator of health; it is useful when used in association with other information about a baby or child.
- **Length/height** is a better long-term indicator of health as it is generally affected only by ill health or a genetic disorder. Children cannot shrink but they can stop growing taller.
- **Head circumference** is the length of the largest circle around

the head; used in conjunction with the other two measurements it is a good indicator of expected growth. In itself it is used to screen for any abnormalities of the brain that cause excessive head growth. It is not measured routinely beyond the first year.

Taking these three measurements allows comparison and indicates that the child is growing properly. Tools of measurement called centile charts have been devised by researching sizes of children of all ages across the UK to give the average expectancy of growth for each age group in both sexes. Copies of the charts are to be found in each child's parent-held record and the health visitor or GP should plot on the charts any measurement taken. They show the child's progress, which is more important than the measurement itself.

What are centile lines?

The 50th centile is the middle dark line. This is the average, the most common size. Any centile below the 50th means smaller than average and any centile above means bigger than average. For example, a child growing on the 10th centile will be among the shortest in the class at school while another growing on the 90th centile will be among the tallest.

The areas below the 2nd centile and above the 98th centile are shaded in order to highlight the necessity to monitor and possibly investigate any measurement in these sections. A measurement below or above the outer limits of the shading indicates the boundaries of what is considered to be an acceptable growth pattern and may similarly need further investigation. Initially, the baby or child may be referred to the GP for assessment and then to a paediatrician.

It is important to remember that these centile charts are only guidelines for assessing growth. It does not matter so much which centile line the child is following, as long as it is roughly the same one. It is not uncommon, however, for babies to move across the lines during the first year, and many older children will also deviate from these limits but will be found to give no cause for concern. For instance, the reason for a baby being small may turn out to be that the baby's parent are small. Only occasionally will a condition that affects growth be uncovered, but early detection of this is of prime importance in order for treatment to be effective.

(NB: The centile charts discussed here are the revised and updated [1995] ones. In the old version the outer limits were the 3rd centile and the 97th centile. The 3rd centile is still sometimes referred to by professionals and books.)

Concerns about weight

Babies are first weighed at birth, and usually quite often in the first few weeks of life, by the midwife and then the health visitor. If a child has any health problem that may affect his weight, (if, for example, he was premature), weighing once a week will probably be recommended for a time but it will really depend on each child.

Some people argue that weighing serves only to increase anxiety in new parents. Breastfeeding mothers may be more concerned about weight as they cannot measure how much milk their baby is drinking and a low weight gain can undermine their confidence in breastfeeding. Breastfed babies can, however, put on weight erratically so it is important to check that the baby is latched on properly, breastfeeding effectively and contented between feeds. For bottle-fed babies, it is easy to calculate that a baby is getting the right amount of milk. In both cases a continued low weight gain with no obvious cause should be checked out by your GP.

Most first-time parents usually find it useful to visit the clinic weekly for the first six weeks or so; weighing the baby is a good starting point for discussing any other concerns. It also gives the health visitor the opportunity to talk about the next stages. The health visitor or GP would let you know if there was any reason for your child to be weighed or measured more frequently; otherwise, it is enough for the child to be routinely weighed and measured at the developmental assessments (see below).

Childhood development

Right from the beginning a healthy child becomes able to do more and more things and adapts better and better to his or her surroundings. Development can be broken down into four main areas.

- **Gross motor** – large body movements e.g. progression from sitting to standing.
- **Fine motor and vision** – control of hand movements combined with visual ability, e.g. progression from holding a large

toy with the whole hand to picking up small objects with the finger and thumb.

- **Speech and hearing** – e.g. responding to sounds and language, an increase in vocabulary, forming sentences.
- **Social behaviour** – the child's ability to look after himself or herself and relate to other people, e.g. progression from playing alone to playing with other children.

How can parents tell whether their child is developing normally?

'Normal' is a difficult word to use of human beings as our wide range of skills and abilities gives us large scope to be different from each other. It is likely that some common ground would be found between two children of the same age, whatever their ability or disability, but many things will be different. Who can say which child is 'normal'? Just as it is impossible to have one expected weight for every age, children will learn to do things at different rates. They tend to be described as being within normal limits of development for their age.

Parents are usually the first to notice any problem with their child's development either by intuition, reading or comparing them with other children of the same age. The following guide will help you to ensure that your child is developing appropriately within the first three years, when development is at its fastest. The ages are guidelines only and correspond to the routine developmental assessments. If you have any concerns discuss them with your health visitor or GP.

Newborn

Large movements

- No voluntary control of movements.
- Arms and legs should all move spontaneously with equal strength.
- Head flops forward or back if not supported.
- Equipped with several 'primitive' reflexes (automatic responses):
  Moro or startle reflex – extends arms then brings them into chest at a sudden noise or if head support is taken away unexpectedly (never do this yourself)
  Grasp reflex – puts hand around finger or object placed against palm
  Stepping reflex – when held securely upright with feet on a surface takes steps as if walking

Rooting reflex – turns head sideways if touched on the side of the cheek near the mouth and tries to suck the object

Sucking reflex – begins to suck on anything placed in the mouth.

Fine movements and vision

- No control over hand movements, only reflex action.
- Vision mainly blurred, the best distance for seeing is about 25cm – the distance between a mother's face and her baby's when the baby is being held or fed.
- Prefers to look at contrast colours, e.g. black and white or bright objects such as the light or windows.
- Shows much interest in the human face.

Speech and hearing

- Startled reaction to loud or sudden noises.
- Hearing can be tested by using electrode equipment but as they get older, babies will wriggle about too much for this equipment to work.
- Cries to indicate hunger, tiredness, a dirty nappy, feeling cold, feeling hot, tummy ache, illness, wants comfort or just generally fed up. This cry could be described as a survival mechanism to ensure that the baby is looked after. Parents and particularly mothers find that they are tuned into the sound of their own baby's cry and while others around them can ignore the crying, parents seem to have the urge to go to the baby.
- Having one cry for all problems makes communication between the baby and the parents difficult in the first weeks of life but over this time the first signs of real communication develop. The mother of a 6-week-old baby will often describe her baby's crying to a visitor as a 'hungry cry' or a 'tired cry' or similarly be concerned that the baby is unwell by saying 'that's not the normal cry'. This is a two-way process. The baby is communicating more effectively using tone and pitch of cry and the mother has tuned into her own baby's signals.
- Makes various noises, moves mouth but with little control.

Social behaviour

- Makes eye contact if face held at about 25cm from another face.
- Will begin to make body movements and changes shape of face

when looking at a person or something of interest such as a bright light to show excitement or concentration.
- Sleeps for most of the time between feeds.

Six-eight weeks
Large movements

- Primitive movements still large and jerky, little control.
- Reflexes still present.
- More head control but not complete.

Fine movements and vision

- Squint (where one eye points into the middle) may be visible but this is common and often corrects itself.
- Continues to prefer near faces and objects.
- Will fix on an object and follow briefly.
- Blink reflex present – closes both eyes to bright light.

Speech and hearing

- Still startled by sudden or loud noise.
- May move eyes towards sound source.
- Usually stops crying and turns towards nearby voice unless very distressed.
- Makes sounds in throat and coos when content and in response to faces or voices.
- Crying more selectively for different reasons.

Social behaviour

- Responsive smiling begins; before this any smiles are usually attributed to wind. This is very encouraging to parents: after six weeks of usually hard work their baby suddenly starts smiling at them. It seems as if the baby knows that his parents are feeling worn out and need some encouragement.
- The baby is awake for longer periods between feeds without crying and can be distracted more easily.

Seven-nine months
Large movements

- Sits with back straight and head firm; may sit alone.

- Takes some or all weight when held standing.
- Holds arms up to be lifted.
- Lifts legs and grasps foot, then puts foot in mouth.
- May attempt to crawl, often backwards first.
- Rolls over both ways.
- Moves around the room by some means, e.g. rolling, shuffling, crawling.
- May pull self up to stand on furniture or reach up and grab things.

Fine movements and vision

- Will look around at anything that attracts the attention, not always preferring people to objects.
- Picks up toys with whole hand (palmar grasp); can pass the toy from one hand to another and study it.
- Beginning to use finger and thumb (pincer grip) to pick up small objects.
- Looks for falling toy and locates it (great game!).

Speech and hearing

- Listens to everyday sounds with interest.
- Makes easy babble sounds like ba-ba and da-da for own amusement and to amuse others.
- Recognises familiar voices and turns quickly.
- Laughs and chuckles, enjoys repetitive games.
- Imitates sounds such as smacking lips or blowing raspberries.
- Beginning to recognise tones of voice – may become upset at a stern 'no' but cannot yet understand that 'no' means 'stop', so this is not an effective method of preventing accidents. Removing the child from danger or offering an interesting toy will be more successful.
- Screams in annoyance or frustration.

Social behaviour

- Puts everything to the mouth.
- Holds and chews finger foods.
- Tries to grab spoon when being fed.
- Becomes rigid and throws head back when cross. This is partic-

ularly evident when changing the nappy at this age as there are far more interesting things for the baby to be doing.

- Enjoys games such as peek-a-boo and clapping hands.
- Will find a toy partly or wholly hidden under a cloth that previously would have been quickly forgotten about. This is an important stage: the baby is now understanding that objects are still there even if they cannot be seen. This may go some way to explaining the fact that at about this time babies become more 'clingy' and cry when their mother or father leave the room. They now understand that if their mother leaves the room she is somewhere else and crying may bring her back.
- Also at this time babies become increasingly wary of unfamiliar people and show a definite preference for their main caregivers. They might even show reluctance to be comforted by their fathers or grandparents – this development can happen over a very short space of time. It can be a difficult time for all concerned but it is an important stage where the baby is exploring his feelings and beginning to realise that he is a separate person. There is no malice in his actions, nor is it a denial of love or a criticism of care. The baby is just sorting out who is important in his life and naturally this will begin with the person he spends most time with.

ATTENTION

Several key stages of development at this age open your baby up to all sorts of danger. He can now move around the room, reach anything on the floor, has control to pick up the tiniest objects and pull down larger, higher-up objects. It is a good idea to get down on the floor and see what your baby can see. Move as much as possible out of the way and use safety equipment where necessary. Your health visitor can help if you need advice. Prepare your house before your baby reaches these key stages. Remember that babies do not understand danger at this age – they only want to explore their world.

Eighteen months

Large movements

- Walks safely alone and can hold toys while walking, and begins to run without bumping into things.
- Pushes and pulls toys and furniture.
- Walks upstairs and maybe down with hand held, usually crawls down backwards.
- Can bend down and pick up toys without losing balance.
- Very good at climbing – safety alert, so needs a safe environment.

Fine movements and vision

- Enjoys picture books, points at familiar objects.
- Holds pen with whole hand, and sometimes makes circular scribble but not for long; may show a preference for using one hand.
- Uses neat pincer grip to pick up tiny objects; usually finds anything the vacuum cleaner has missed.
- Looks with interest at people or cars and so on in the distance or out of the window.

Speech and hearing

- Chatters away to self imitating the sound of a conversation but without real words.
- Uses 7+ recognisable words.
- Understands simple sentences and instructions.
- Listens to sounds and conversation but attention span short.
- Communicates needs by pointing and vocalising.
- Enjoys singing and music, and tries to join in.
- Points to body parts when prompted by someone else.

Social behaviour

- Feeds self, enjoys mess.
- Can remove clothes but not put them on.
- Still prefers familiar people.
- Enjoys copying adult behaviour like vacuuming and washing up.
- Tends to know what he wants and can usually remember where to find it.

- May understand that 'no' means 'stop' but hates to be stopped, demonstrates annoyance by screaming, punching and kicking. Saying 'no' is still not a reliable method of preventing accidents as at this age as children are beginning to test their boundaries and will see how far they can go. Physical restraint is usually required near roads, ponds etc.
- Gets involved with games such as putting toys in and out of containers; will play on own for some time but becomes anxious if he loses sight of the familiar adult.
- May indicate when nappy is wet or dirty, may know when he is actually going.

Three years
Large movements

- Walks up and down stairs safely.
- Walks in all directions and can pull large objects, beginning to recognise own strength.
- Can stand on one foot and maybe hop, may walk on tiptoe.
- Runs around safely and enjoys jumping and climbing.

Fine movements and vision

- Can thread large beads.
- Has good control of pencil in preferred hand, holds it between finger and thumb, can copy a circle, beginning to draw recognisable faces and other objects.
- May know names of colours and be able to match them.
- Recognises images of tiny people in photos.
- Paints with large brush and cuts with some control of scissors.

Speech and hearing

- Enjoys and concentrates on stories, knows favourites.
- Speech includes an ever-growing vocabulary; can carry out simple conversation and can describe events though he may not always want to when questioned.
- Can sing several nursery rhymes.
- Speech usually understood by everyone though much of the pronunciation and grammar is not correct; familiar adults rarely misunderstand but it is at this stage that it is important to repeat

the correct sentence so that the child will learn properly.
- Asks repeated questions until there are no more answers!

Social behaviour

- Enjoys helping adults.
- Enjoys many different types of play including make-believe and floor play and will happily play alone or join in with other children.
- Beginning to understand the concept of sharing though can still be jealous of a parent's attention to sibling.
- Feeds self with fork and spoon and is safe with a drink.
- Usually dry in the day, but still needs reminding to go to the toilet as reluctant to interrupt play; may be dry at night but usually still in a nappy. It is not abnormal for a child of three to be wearing nappies all the time.
- More reliable in understanding danger and usually can understand why things are happening but still can become upset if stopped.
- Does not like to be made fun of and will remember everything he or she hears – beware!
- Still shy of strangers but can usually be won round quite easily, so teach wariness of strangers.

Routine assessments

Each child undergoes routine health assessments; what happens at these varies to some extent from health authority to health authority, so what follows is a general guideline. The involvement of the health visitor and the doctor (whether the GP or the community doctor) at each stage of the developmental checks may also vary.

- **Birth:** in hospital by paediatrician (or at home by the GP if a home delivery); consists of physical examination.
- **Six-eight weeks:** at the surgery by GP; consists of physical examination and discussion about feeding etc. and any parental concerns.
- **Seven-nine months:** a distraction test, which although imprecise as a hearing test is a good screening test and developmental assessment; it is carried out at the surgery or clinic by the health

visitor or doctor with an assistant. The check should also include discussion about feeding, sleeping etc. and any other parental concerns (see also below).

- **Eighteen-twenty-four months**: developmental assessment at home, clinic or surgery with the health visitor or the doctor (see also below).
- **Three-four years**: developmental assessment at home, clinic or surgery by   the health visitor, possibly in conjunction with the community doctor or GP.
- **School entry**: physical examination (height, weight, heart; also testes in boys) by community doctor, and/or hearing and eye test by school nurse; all performed at school.

There are also routine **physical examinations** at the ages of 7-8, 11-12 and 14. These are undertaken by doctors and include listening to the heart, asking about hearing, and checking the vision, the hips and all the reflexes; checking that the testes have descended in boys; and looking for any sign of a congenital abnormality.

The 7-9 month hearing test

Before the age of 7-9 months the baby is not developed enough to be tested and after this time it is impossible to tell whether a child is responding to sound or simply playing, so the timing of the test is significant. The test appears basic but anyone performing a hearing test must have completed some special training. If there is any doubt about a child's hearing the test will be repeated; if doubt continues at the second test the child will be referred to the specialist hearing clinic. Many children who are referred are found not to have any hearing problem but early identification of any defect will greatly improve the child's chances of speech and social development.

The 18-24-month developmental assessment

This usually involves a set of toys designed specifically to assess different areas of child development. The person conducting the test will try to get the child to do certain things with the toys or will just watch the child playing with them. He or she will also to listen to any concern raised by a parent about the child's development and follow this up.

Research similar to that carried out to monitor child growth has identified expected limits of development in each area and age group, and various charts have been drawn up for professionals to use alongside their own experience of assessing many children at different ages. The developmental assessments are useful because parents and professionals can discuss the child's development and identify any potential problems or confirm that no problem seems to exist. The parents bring an in-depth knowledge of their child to the assessment and the professional brings an in-depth knowledge of child development.

Often parents are concerned that their child has not done well in the assessment because he or she does not like strangers or is having a bad day. This concern is misplaced as such behaviour is common; the professional will simply ask you questions about what your child normally does at home. There is no need for the child to 'perform' and no mark is given.

What happens if a problem is identified?

The person carrying out the assessment will discuss it with you and either refer your child to an appropriate specialist or decide to review your child again in the near future. For example, it is very common after the 18-month assessment for a health visitor to review a child's speech again at two years, perhaps because he or she is saying only a couple of real words. If parents were particularly concerned about a child's speech or development, the health visitor might decide to refer the child to the GP, a speech therapist or the community doctor. This will mean another appointment and assessment but whoever is involved will be able to give you advice about how to encourage your child's development and decide on any treatment necessary.

Children with special needs

Children found to have a problem that will reduce their educational abilities are said to have special needs. Problems range from potentially complex physical or learning disabilities such as cerebral palsy, Down's Syndrome and autism to any significant hearing, vision or speech defect.

Once a problem like this is suspected or identified, the child should be referred to a specialist unit. This unit is usually found within the local hospital and consists of a team of professionals headed by a paediatric consultant. The team should be able to provide the various therapies that the child needs, as well as information about any diagnosis and potential problems. The family will also have access to a social worker who can advise on support agencies, financial help, local parent networks and funding for any respite care. As well as this service many areas have voluntary agencies who work specifically with children with special needs and their families.

The local authority has an obligation to provide services to enable children with special needs to reach their full potential under the 1989 Children Act. If the child is found to have such a problem the local education authority should be notified by the consultant so that the child can undergo a full assessment by members of health, social and educational services. The aim of the assessment is to look at the child's needs as a whole and involve the family as much as possible. The assessment will conclude with a *Statement of Educational Needs* for the child. This process is known as 'statementing' and can take many months. The aims are to identify what type of educational help the child will need and to secure the necessary funding.

Once this process has been completed, there may be another long wait before a way of meeting the child's needs is identified and funding is agreed. The earlier this process begins, the better for the child. Parents should make their views about their child's needs known, and consider issues such as attendance at mainstream or special schools.

Other parents who have been through this process can be a great help. There is a national register of children with different syndromes and conditions so that parents can contact other parents with children who have the same diagnosis. This can be accessed via the health visitor or social worker. Most areas also have local parent groups to support parents through the statementing process, which can be daunting and confusing. Health visitors, social workers and school nurses can also be called upon for support and advice.

The importance of play

For children, to play is to learn. Humans and many animals learn by doing, by trial and error, by repeating activities again and again until they have understood or mastered the activity. It is their main way of learning before they acquire language. Children can play on their own, with other people, quietly or energetically, and this variety is important for different areas of their development. A child that is never left alone to play will probably get as frustrated as a child who is always left alone.

Children are naturally inquisitive and will play with anything around them. This is why if you give a baby a yoghurt and a spoon the yoghurt will go everywhere. The baby may have the skill to get the yoghurt into the mouth but will find it more interesting to explore what the yoghurt does on the table. First it's a blob, then, if a hand goes into it, it makes a pattern and looks bigger; now there's some on the hand – it feels wet and Mum says: 'What a mess!' Is this what a mess looks like? Now Mum puts the cloth over the yoghurt and the yoghurt disappears – where has it gone?

As you can see there are endless possibilities for learning in this situation. Once the baby has learnt everything he can from it he may eat the yoghurt, and may also learn that food is for eating, or he may learn that if he makes a mess he gets your attention, so this is a good way of getting your attention. In this case there may be certain rules you want your child to learn; remember that children learn by repetition, so if you decide on a rule stick to it; try not to chop and change as this will confuse the child. Consistency is a key word that keeps coming up repeatedly when dealing with children. It particularly applies to children with behavioural or emotional problems – see Chapter 6.

Toys teach children shapes and colours and so on, but many similar items can be made at home very simply. Young children are not fussy. It is usually through school contacts that children become socialised into wanting particular makes and models of toys so make the most of the pre-school years to save money. An activity gym for a baby and a tea-set for a toddler will provide hours of entertainment and learning. Most areas also have a toy library from which you can borrow toys. A weekly visit to the library will be something children look forward to and it's free. *Creative Play* by Dorothy Einon (Penguin, 1985) suggests play ideas for children from 0 to 10.

Playgroups and nurseries are very important for children's development and preparation for school. First try taking your child to a mother and toddler group where he or she will learn certain social skills. From two-and-a-half to three years start him or her at a play group. Many schools now have nursery departments. This will give the child some stimulating activity the year before starting school and it is free. Health visitors have up-to-date lists of local playgroups, mother and toddler groups as well as private nurseries.

Quality time

'Quality time' is a current buzzphrase used mainly in the context of parents who are out at work all day. It suggests that the quality of time spent with children is more important than the quantity of time spent with them. It also seems to suggest that the parent needs to do something wonderful during this time. However, children do not usually need to be shown how to play – they are experts. The parent's role is to ensure that children have opportunities to play and to encourage and listen to their child's achievements. Whether you are out working or at home with the distractions of normal family life 'quality time' can simply be seen as giving your child some attention, such as reading a story, playing in the bath or just listening to what he has to say. The simplest way to encourage a child's development is to talk to him from birth onwards. It does not matter what you say. At first he won't understand but he will begin to learn the art of conversation.

Watching television

There is no doubt that some television is educational for a child. It also gives children the opportunity to relax, as much of their day's play is busy and requires concentration, and gives parents a break from close supervision. It is a good idea, however, to limit the amount of television a child watches. Children can become transfixed by the television and it stops them exploring the rest of their abilities. For young children you may want to limit it to periods when they are tired or when you need to do something like cook the tea or early in the morning to stop them waking up the household. They will happily watch the same video numerous times, so it is a good idea if you have a video recorder to tape some programmes so that children can watch them at a time that suits you. For older children, you could limit television-watching to a particular time so that they learn to be selective in what they watch. Many families now watch television at mealtimes; this is an automatic block to conversation and children miss out on learning this social skill.

Using computers

Computers are undoubtedly being used more and more at school, and it may therefore be an advantage to have one at home. Time spent at the computer is a sedentary and solitary activity and may reduce the chance of children exploring other areas of play so, as with television, it is probably worth limiting. Computer games are addictive, and although they require some skill in concentration, visual acuity and dexterity, they have little further value other than to occupy the child's time. They may even be considered harmful to the development of children, particularly younger ones, by stopping them engaging in more constructive play.

Against this, if properly used computers can be a useful educational tool. It is important that children do have some exposure to computers at an early age. As with television and videos, the use of the computer – and the Internet – and the time spent using it should be carefully monitored by parents; and likewise, computers are useful aids but no substitute for playing and talking and interacting with other children.

Why is exercise important?

Exercise helps children develop strong muscles, grow, develop good lung capacity, use up excess energy, encourages good sleeping patterns, and gives people a healthy start to life. It is also important for setting good habits for adulthood, so reducing the risk of heart disease and other chronic problems such as obesity.

Evidence shows that children have become progressively less active over the past 20 years. Babies and young children are naturally active but they must be given opportunities to exercise. A baby who is always left in his cot will not be able to explore much and will lose incentive to move. Similarly, a toddler who stays in only one room watching the television may not be motivated to exercise. A baby that is put on the floor with toys all around will be encouraged to move and a toddler taken to the park will run around and jump all over the equipment. Sedentary activities should be balanced with opportunities for exercise such as walks, using swings and going swimming. Walk to school with your child, if it is near enough and safe to do so.

Many parents are reluctant to allow children out of the house without an adult because of fears relating to crime, drugs and abduction. Twenty years ago children ran around on open spaces and parks with friends and especially in the summer it was hard to keep them in. Today's security considerations put greater demands on the parents to supervise their children. Consider taking it in turns to share this responsibility with a group of other parents.

Common problems

Some aspects of the following areas are also covered in the A–Z starting on page 146 – see the index for further leads. See also Chapter 6.

Sleep problems

Sleep is one of the most common topics for discussion between parents and health visitors and although every parent feels totally alone when sitting with a wide-awake baby in the middle of the night, thousands of other bleary-eyed parents are awake too, wondering why they ever decided to have children.

The early months

The most common time for wakeful nights is in the first three months of a baby's life. Some babies sleep through the night from the beginning while others will wake frequently; this may be just the luck of the draw but there is a belief that a traumatic delivery can affect a baby's sleep and crying pattern. If you think that this might be the case you can visit a cranio-osteopath. Over a course of several sessions the osteopath gently manipulates the head to correct any damaged nerve pathways. (A fee is usually charged but may be waived if you are claiming benefit.)

It is advisable to encourage a sense of day and night for the baby so at night keep the lights low and try not to play with the baby or make too much noise, keep activity to a minimum, and change the nappy only if it is dirty or very wet. You may have to accept that you are going to be woken in the night for several weeks or months and adapt your life accordingly – try to sleep in the day while the baby sleeps, or ask someone to babysit while you sleep. You may have to adjust your routine for a while so that you go to bed at 9 o'clock as this is when your baby sleeps for four hours. Hang on to the fact that this situation will not last for ever. If you are tired cut down on activities during the day, keep housework to the essentials, and fill the freezer with ready-made meals. Accept that you are going to be tired for a while and give yourself as easy a time as you can.

From about three to six months babies may still want one or two feeds in the night even though they don't necessarily need it. If your baby is still feeding more than this at night and you are finding it difficult talk to your health visitor.

Six months onwards

From six months feeding in the night is not necessary and is done only out of habit. If your baby's or child's waking is becoming a problem you should be able to do something about it. Tackling a sleep problem is, however, always easier said than done. The theory of knowing how to solve the problem is not always enough and can cause more stress if not carried out correctly. It is advisable therefore to seek professional support from your health visitor; in some areas special sleep clinics have been set up.

Sleep is only a problem if it is affecting the child or family. A child who is waking at night may display difficult behaviour during the day. This can be what the parent focuses on as a problem, when in fact if the child's sleep improved so might his behaviour the next day. Alternatively, the child's waking may be focused on as the problem by a parent who is experiencing a stressful time at work, when in fact if the work-related stress were reduced the parent might manage the child's waking better.

These sorts of issues will affect how you tackle the problem and how successful you are likely to be. This is why it is useful to seek individual advice and support from someone who can help look at the whole picture of family life objectively and so help you choose the right approach.

The 'controlled crying technique'

There are no one-sentence miracle answers to sleep problems but a common method that works well with babies over six months old is known as the 'controlled crying technique', which involves allowing your baby to cry. Many parents find it hard to think of attempting it until a certain point when they know they have just got to get some sleep themselves.

The parent returns every 5–10 minutes to repeat the same goodnight words, with no cuddles, just to reassure the baby that the parent has not abandoned him (though this will not make the baby any less angry) and reassure the parent that the baby is not in danger. The aim is for the baby to have no incentive to stay awake for the next parental visit.

If you try this for an hour and then give up and pick up the baby to rock him to sleep you will both feel stressed and the baby will only learn to cry longer next time. This is why it is important to prepare yourself and feel committed – in fact, do not attempt this method unless you feel strong enough to persevere, otherwise it will only be an upsetting waste of time. It is also important not to tackle the problem when the child is unwell or teething as this is not fair on the child and will be unlikely to work. If you *do* decide to try it:

- Ensure the baby has had enough to eat and drink, is clean and comfortable and is not too hot or too cold.
- Put the baby in the cot awake, and make him comfortable.
- Look at him and say in a calm but firm voice something like: 'Mummy/Daddy loves you but it is time to go to sleep now. I'll be next door/downstairs. Good night.'
- Turn away and walk out of the room.
- This is where your heartstrings will be pulled as a desperate cry will now be let rip. This is a cry of anger at your leaving and frustration at not having the usual comfort.
- Go as far away as possible, do something to keep busy, turn up the volume on the television or music, or go into the garden.
- Time five minutes; if the baby is still crying, go back in. Repeat the same lines and don't pick up the baby but make him comfortable as quickly as possible. If the child is older and standing up, lie him back down and tuck him in.
- Leave the room, and time another five minutes. Continue this sequence until the baby is asleep. The five-minute period can be lengthened to 10–15 minutes when you feel more comfortable about what you are doing.

Remember: you are aiming for your return to the bedroom to be as boring as possible, so the baby has no incentive to stay awake for your next arrival. Note also that just leaving a baby to cry alone for half an hour is not using this technique as he is getting no reassurance from you, so may be feeling alone and scared.

This technique is described here in its basic form. The approach can be softened by involving some form of comfort but it should be less than the baby is used to, such as the parent merely staying in the room rather than actually holding the baby.

The longest sleep will be sustained by encouraging your child to go to sleep in the cot without any comfort such as a feed, a dummy, music or rocking. This is because during the night sleep varies from deep to light. During the light sleep periods we are almost awake. If a baby or young child is only used to getting to sleep with some form of comfort, then in his light sleep phases he will realise that the comfort is not there and be unable to settle back into deep sleep without it, so he will wake up and cry. Like any habit it can be tough to break.

Solving a child's night waking can have a dramatic effect on your life but you have to be very committed to solving it for it to work. Focus on the benefits to the family. Carefully pick the right time to tackle it, when you have a few days off from work or when a relative can be around in the day so that you can catch up on your sleep. Warn your neighbours so that they can move rooms if necessary. If you cannot face trying at night try it during the day if your child has a nap. Parents are often surprised at how little time it actually takes to break the pattern – often just two or three nights and only short periods of crying – but prepare yourself for a week of wakeful nights. It is worth trying to tackle a sleep problem at a young age as it is harder when children get older and therefore more mobile and vocal.

Once you have been sucessful at breaking the habit of night waking your child may revert to it during periods of illness or disruption to the usual routine. You should however find it easier to tackle again once the child is back to normal.

Toilet training

Physical control of the bowel using the nervous system is not usually present until about 18 months or more and control of the

ENCOURAGING GOOD SLEEPING HABITS

- Stop using a dummy in the day.
- Put your baby to sleep in quiet, darkened room during the day from birth, even if he is sleeping in your room at night.
- You may want to leave a light on in the hall or use a glow plug in the child's room.
- Try not to start using rocking or music as methods of getting a child to sleep.
- Crying is often a sign of tiredness in children and leaving them on their own to cry for a few minutes may release their tension and so help them to get to sleep – always check them quietly after a few minutes or after they go quiet.
- Bath, drink, teeth, story, sleep and a regular bedtime help to prepare a child for the night. In other words, establish a regular routine which culminates in going to bed.
- Baby massage can help to relax a baby for the night.
- Letting children nap in the day (not after about 3 o'clock) will often help them to sleep at night.
- Ensure that your child has had enough to eat during the day and make sure that he has had some exercise.
- Make sure that no bright street light or any regular night noises such as those of water system disturb your child's sleep.
- Make sure the child is not too hot or too cold. Touching the back of a baby's neck with the back of your hand will give a good indication of his temperature. Don't be fooled by cold hands or feet – this is due to poor circulation and not body temperature. Always follow the guidelines on temperature control in line with reducing the risk of cot death (see page 39). Nursery thermometers are available with markings for optimum temperatures.
- Sleep often becomes a problem when children are teething or ill; see the GP to reassure yourself, and give your child paracetamol syrup if he has a temperature or is complaining of pains. Try homeopathic remedies for teething and minor ailments to help him sleep.
- Older children may be encouraged not to wake you in the morning by having a clock by their bed and being told to stay in bed until the little hand reaches a particular time (only for children who can be trusted to be awake in the house without adult supervision).
- There will always be times when tired parents feel that measures such as bringing their child into bed with them are the only way of coping. If you do this, just try not to let it develop into a habit.

bladder follows about six months later. Toilet training can occur younger than this: for example, in countries where disposable nappies are difficult to obtain babies may learn bladder and bowel control sooner for their own comfort. With disposable nappies, children have much less incentive to control themselves.

It is normal for a child to become toilet-trained during the day any time between eighteen months and three years. It will depend, like most such attainments, on the child, the parents and the family situation, as well as an element of luck.

Try to keep pressure about toilet-training to a minimum, not forgetting how stubborn children of this age can be. Get your child used to having a potty around and sitting on it before toilet-training even starts. Let your child see you sitting on the toilet. Go with your child's pace when you do start the training, and give lots of praise for sitting on the potty, and more for a result. Don't be cross about accidents – children can still have an accident up to the age of seven – and the younger the child, the more reminders he or she will need, especially when engrossed in play.

If the plan doesn't seem to be working and you are feeling stressed stop trying and leave it completely for three months. It's usually better to have a go in the summer as there are fewer clothes to wash. Night-time dryness usually takes a bit longer as the bladder cannot always hold nine or more hours' worth of urine. Seek advice from your health visitor, school nurse or GP if you are unhappy with your child's progress.

Bedwetting

All young babies are incontinent during the day and at night. Many children are dry during the day by the age of three but are still wet at night. Boys take longer to control their bladder than girls. By the age of five most children are completely dry both during the day and night. Even so, there is still a significant minority who wet their beds at night; many health authority areas do not treat night-time bedwetting until the age of seven. The technical name for this is **nocturnal enuresis**. Sometimes there may be a physical reason, such as a kidney problem, or it may simply be a case of slow development. Occasionally, children can become wet again after being dry for some time. This could be the result of a stressful event such as a new addition to the family, discord at home or at school or the death of a relative such as a grandparent.

If you are worried by your child's night-time wetting discuss it with the health visitor, school nurse or your GP. The doctor may wish to feel the child's tummy and make sure that no obvious abnormality exists. This is unlikely but should be checked all the same. Equally, a sample of urine should be checked too by dipping chemical sticks into it to make sure it has no abnormal contents such as sugar or protein. The same sample should be sent to the lab to exclude the possibility of infection. If there is any doubt an ultrasound scan – the same type as that given to pregnant women – will be performed to examine the kidneys and the bladder.

Assuming that all is well, the vast majority of bed-wetters will eventually settle down and be dry both during the day and the night. By the time adolescence is reached only about 1 per cent may have problems with bladder control. Even so this can be a distressing symptom which deserves serious consideration.

The use of star charts works well with some children. Explain to the child that each time he has a dry night he can stick a star on a chart, and that when he has gained a certain number of stars he will be rewarded by a particular gift.

Regular emptying of the bladder during the day and putting the child on the toilet late in the evening may help, but the late evening visits may be disturbing to a child woken from sleep.

A 'buzzer' may help: this consists of a detector pad which is placed under the bottom sheet and the unit is powered by a battery. As the child begins to pass urine, the alarm sounds and wakes the child, who should then stop passing urine, get up and go to the toilet. Such units can be bought by mail order or borrowed from health visitors or community clinics. Success rates are surprisingly good.

Drugs don't cure the problem but can give temporary relief. They may be suitable for the older child who is going away for a while to stay with a relative or friend or going on a school trip. The tablets available are potentially very dangerous if taken as an overdose so should be stored in a safe place far from inquisitive hands. There is also a nasal spray which can be effective. Both types of medication are available only on prescription from your doctor.

Herbal medicine and homeopathy may also have something to offer, and counselling in a co-operative older child may make a valuable contribution to solving the problem.

Soiling

Most children can be considered 'clean' by about the age of 2; not to have attained bowel control by the age of four would be considered abnormal – you should seek professional help from your health visitor or GP. Just like bed-wetting, delayed bowel control is commoner in boys than in girls and is often just a sign of slower development.

As with bed-wetting, children with emotional or stressful problems are more at risk of having problems controlling their bowels. Some children develop a reluctance to have their bowels open, causing constipation problems. Some use the situation to exert control over their parents, but it may happen simply because they have experienced pain when having their bowels open in the past. This problem is quite difficult to manage and requires sensitive handling in order not to worsen the problem – seek advice from your health visitor or GP.

Another not uncommon problem is that young children develop a fear about having their bowels open on the toilet and insist on putting on a nappy. This fear can be difficult to dislodge but if they are not pressurised into using the toilet it may resolve itself. An older child of four upwards may require some help from a child psychologist.

Occasionally children deliberately deposit fully formed faecal material in an inappropriate and unacceptable place – this is called **encopresis**. This kind of behaviour may be difficult to stop and may need expert psychiatric help.

Crying

Crying is a powerful means of communication. Babies vary widely in their crying patterns: some cry occasionally while others cry incessantly. One of the main functions of crying is to alert the carers to a problem but to start with there may be no clue as to the cause. However, as parents get to know their baby, they may start to understand what makes the baby more likely to cry. Even so, sometimes they can be stumped. Try working through this checklist.

- **Hunger**: perhaps the first thought. If the baby has just been fed, a small top-up feed may settle him, but be careful – if the baby is feeding frequently or if he is colicky more food will make it worse. Sometimes babies can get into a cycle of having small and frequent feeds and so do not feel full for long. If the baby will stop crying to suck a clean finger or dummy he is not starving. Soothe him in this way for as long as possible – he will then take a more substantial feed next time and settle for longer.

- **Wind**: a common complaint, suggested if the baby has been fed, fallen asleep but begins to fidget and wake as soon as he has been laid down. He will stop crying when put upright.
- **Nappy needs changing**: the baby may be unhappy with a dirty nappy or may even be suffering from the effects of a nappy rash.
- **Colic**: no one knows exactly what colic is but it certainly gives babies a lot of pain in their tummies. It may occur up to the age of three or four months and is most common in the evening. It is characterised by the baby screaming and drawing up the legs Hang on to the fact that it will pass.
- **Cold**: babies prefer being warm to being cold – this is why they often cry when they are undressed. On the other hand many new parents make the mistake of wrapping their babies too warmly, especially indoors, which makes them uncomfortable.
- **Tiredness**: babies get easily tired and react by crying.
- **Teething**: always a likely cause in an unhappy baby but not always easy to prove.
- **Ill health**: crying may be the first or even the only sign that there is something physically wrong with the baby.
- **No apparent reason**: after running through the checklist, there may still be no obvious cause. If it's a new symptom and out of character don't feel awkward about taking the baby to the doctor for a check-up, particularly if the crying persists. Even then it is possible that no specific cause will be identified. Remember that a bout of crying on its own is unlikely to do the baby any harm.

Coping

Just as some babies are more likely to cry than others some parents are more able to cope with it than others. A parent with a supportive partner, with experience of other children and with a good network of friends and family nearby is more likely to cope than someone who is more isolated. Even so, constant crying can be wearing, causing tensions in the family. Once it has been recognised as a problem, it is important for the family, particularly the main carer, to develop coping mechanisms.

Assuming you have eliminated all the obvious possible causes of distress then there are certain things that may help. Plain and simple contact with your baby by holding him or her close to you, perhaps in a sling or against your shoulder, may help. Wrapping in a shawl – swaddling – is a well-established calming technique, the theory being that it reminds babies of the womb. In addition, it stops them being upset by their own flailing limb movements. Even if this does not help the baby, it may help soothe you. If the baby falls asleep swaddled make sure that the head is not covered and loosen the shawl before lying him down, as swaddling babies tightly can lead to them overheating.

Even the movement caused by taking your baby on to your shoulder may be sufficient to calm him. Try swaying the baby or rocking him in his pram; and you would not be the first parent to strap the baby in the car and go for a drive.

Massage may work, and it can also be soothing to an anxious parent. Remember to keep the room warm if you are massaging your baby. Use some baby oil to lubricate your fingers and begin by gently stroking the hands and feet. Then move up the limbs while talking softly. Also vary the patterns, such as stroking in circular patterns as well as up and down.

Sucking has a natural calming influence on a baby and you have a choice between a dummy and a thumb. There are various schools of thought on which is the better but the decision may ultimately be the baby's.

The use of sound may be another course of action, such as singing a lullaby, having the television, radio or washing machine droning on. Pre-recorded tapes of soothing music are another possibility.

Many of the methods recommended here contradict advice given for establishing good sleeping habits (see page 78). Each set of parents must weigh up the situation for themselves with their own baby. If the parents are exhausted and the baby is crying, they will be ready to try anything to get the baby to sleep. If your priority is getting rest now, then do whatever you have to in order to settle your baby – you can tackle the problem later when you feel more up to it, and will feel less worried about the crying of an older, more resilient baby. Other parents will feel happier if they have established routines early.

These techniques may not work and may even be counter-productive – after all, excessive stimulation may irritate the baby even more, causing more crying. In this situation it's worth putting the baby in the cot and leaving him to cry for a while. He may just settle. It is also important to do this if you are beginning to feel very angry with your baby for crying. This is understandable but can easily lead to guilt. Make sure the baby is safe in the cot, and then get as far away from him as possible to take five minutes out for a drink and something to eat, or have a cry yourself. When you go back to your baby you will feel more able to cope and realise that the baby is not crying deliberately but trying to communicate discomfort. If your anger does not go away it is very important that you talk to someone.

Talk to your partner and friends and discuss the problem openly. You may be surprised at what other people have had to cope with. Often at this point parents at the end of their tether realise that they are not inadequate after all and that there is no need to feel guilty. Getting out and about with other people often helps to reduce tension and share the burden. Sometimes it's useful to discuss the matter with health professionals, especially the health visitor, who will be seeing you and the baby anyway. She will have had lots of practical experience of dealing with crying babies. Your GP is another person you may want to speak to, but remember that nobody is going to offer you a cure. Self-help groups can be invaluable in providing assistance. The National Childbirth Trust★ has post-natal support groups and CRY-SIS★ provides support for parents of children who cry too much.

You might like to keep a diary to see if a pattern of events is common to crying episodes. If so, it could lead to your adopting a different strategy and at least will help you feel you are doing something positive.

Temper tantrums

These outbursts accompany a natural stage of development and usually begin at around 18 months to two years – hence the term the 'terrible twos'. Some parents think themselves lucky if their child has not displayed this behaviour by three but as this is a natural stage of development, parents may then experience a difficult period with their child at a later age. The temper tantrums of a

2-year-old are particularly disturbing to parents because they involve what appears to be the whole range of the child's physical energy and voice. This makes the child very difficult to handle or ignore in public places and becomes a source of embarrassment.

There are a number of reasons for the tantrums. First, the child is seeing how far he can push you. A child needs to do this and have boundaries; two is an age for a child when there seem to be many barriers and many 'no's. Also, he does not yet fully understand the reasons why he is being stopped, so this leads to a lot of pent-up frustration and anger; at this age children are realising the control they can have over adults and the power of their own strength and voice.

To cope with temper tantrums:

- Decide on your boundaries – rules of behaviour – such as two stories before bed. Try to agree these rules between both parents, and then – this is the hard part – stick to them. Your child will soon learn that it is not worth fighting if you are not going to give in.
- Do not restrict your child unless it is necessary – saying no can become a habit. If your child wants to wear the yellow tee-shirt and you want him to wear the blue, let him choose. If he won't put a coat on to go out, leave it off and take it with you – he'll soon want it if he's cold. If you say no only when it is important he is more likely to understand.
- Praise him when he is good or even just not in a temper. For instance, if he gets round the supermarket without a tantrum give him a hug and say how good he has been. Reward him with a story at home or playing a game. If he gets through the morning without a tantrum do the same – he will soon learn that you are more fun to be with when he does not have tantrums.
- Whenever possible ignore the tantrum. Make sure that he is safe and either turn your back or leave the room. Do the vacuuming to drown the noise, but keep an eye on him in case he changes tactics on getting your attention – part of the reason for the temper is to get your attention; children don't differentiate between negative and positive attention so shouting at them can be just as rewarding for them as praise. If you don't pay any attention the child will soon get bored and want to make friends when you go back to him, but he also might just feel better for getting rid of some anger.

- Consistency is a vital ingredient in managing a tantrum, regardless of the course of action taken. A policy of ignoring the tantrum while ensuring the safety of the child is reasonable as long as you stick to it. Changing tack halfway through a tantrum, perhaps because you feel guilty or you can't cope with the child's distress, may turn out to be a short-term gain at long-term expense.
- If you can see a tantrum looming try distracting your child: if he doesn't want to leave the swings, point to a dog in the distance and suggest that he runs to catch it.
- Try to use bribery with sweets only as a last resort or at times when best behaviour is important – otherwise this creates its own problems.
- Some parents use smacking as a means of disciplining their child. If you do, choose your moment carefully. Repeated smacks will soon lose any effect on discipline. In addition, children will learn by the example set to them, so the wrong conclusion drawn is that smacking or hitting someone is reasonable behaviour.
- Try particularly never to smack in your own anger, but leave the room and count to ten. Even though he's behaving like a monster, the child needs to know that you still love him whatever he may have done, and hitting out in anger will only make you feel guilty later.
- Keep a diary: often it is obvious what has precipitated the crisis but sometimes there may be no clues as to why the child has developed a tantrum. A simple diary of events leading up to a tantrum may identify a cause.
- If you are finding things difficult contact your health visitor and try reading *Toddler Taming: A parent's guide to the first four years* by Dr C. Green (Vermilion, 1992).

Breath-holding attacks

Breath-holding attacks are an extreme form of temper tantrum; they are the child's most dramatic gesture and not surprisingly can reduce parents to immediate acquiescence. They are horrible to witness because the child will actually turn blue and may then lose consciousness. Afterwards the child resumes his normal breathing patterns. Naturally, he receives the attention he wanted and will be encouraged to repeat the exercise. Don't let it become a habit but seek medical advice after the first episode.

Occasionally, prolonged breath-holding can in fact provoke a true epileptic fit. From a medical point of view it is essential that a firm diagnosis is made in case the child is epileptic. Once the diagnosis of breath-holding attacks is established, usually by a paediatrician, the treatment is to be firm and take no action during the attacks, except to ensure the child's safety. Eventually the child will understand that this type of dramatic gesture will not achieve the aim of controlling the parents.

Other areas of expertise of a health visitor

Becoming a parent is perhaps the most challenging role you have had to face. Your relationship with your partner, your parents and your friends is likely to change. Many people are choosing to have children later in life; they feel confident at work and enjoy life but perhaps have become too comfortable, used to doing what they want when they want. So the sudden introduction of a small being that depends on its parents for everything is a great shock to their relationship. They cannot go out as they used to, may find it difficult to manage a meal together or even sleep in the same bed. It is undoubtedly a stressful time when both parents are also tired, which does not help. Before having children, no matter how much friends and family tell you, no one seems to believe how difficult it really is – perhaps it goes back to our human instinct of only learning what we actually experience.

Having a child of your own makes you think of your own childhood and can challenge the way you think about your parents. If you were expecting something from your parents that they were not able to offer you may have become angry. Your parents may not be alive and this may upset you. You may expect your partner to behave in a certain way and he or she does the opposite – this also may make you angry or upset. You and your relationships will adjust to this in time though it may seem difficult at first.

Things that might help

- Talk over problems, but try to pick a time when you are not both exhausted.
- Reduce stress wherever possible: use easy-to-prepare food and

do only essential housework, getting someone else to clear the ironing basket or do the cleaning.
- Take up offers of help from friends and family.
- Plan ahead and talk about views on discipline, education and so on. You may have to compromise but agreeing on these issues will help things go more smoothly.
- Try to see your partner's point of view. It is hard being at home all day with a baby or young child, and it is also hard going to work all day when you have been woken in the night.
- When you have some time together try to make the effort to do something you used to do – don't get bogged down with chores.
- If you are having problems with overbearing parents either talk to them or, if this is too difficult, reduce the time you spend with them by inviting them only at certain times. Take their visit as an opportunity to have a rest or pop to the shops.
- If you had bad experiences as a child it might help to talk to someone; you could speak to your GP or health visitor or, if you prefer someone anonymous, you may want to speak to a counsellor.

Post-natal depression

Post-natal depression is identified when a mother continually feels low after she has had a baby. It can begin gradually or suddenly either soon after the birth or several months later. Women may have a number of conflicting thoughts and feelings about themselves, other people and their baby. It can be difficult for women to talk about these negative feelings at a time that is supposed to be full of joy and celebration. This increases their feelings of isolation and despair. Most parents experience some anger or frustration towards their baby or child at some point; if you are feeling depressed these feelings might be heightened. At least 12 per cent of all new mothers are identified as suffering from post-natal depression and probably more go unnoticed.

Health visitors see many women who suffer some type of depression after having a baby. Most women will begin to feel better by just acknowledging the problem with their GP or health visitor. Being listened to is in itself immensely comforting and health visitors will try to offer you some time just for this. Other professionals such as community psychiatric nurses or counsellors may also be available to help.

Some women may need to take a course of anti-depressants. A course may have to be taken for several months, perhaps longer. Modern anti-depressants are not addictive and are worth trying if recommended by your doctor. If you do have these symptoms it will be hard for both you and your partner, so give your partner information about the depression. Leaflets are available from the Association for Post-Natal Illness.★ It may also be useful for your partner to talk to the health visitor.

Things that might help

- Talk to your partner about how you are feeling.
- Talk to your GP or health visitor.
- Rest as much as possible.
- Try to get out of the house, even if only down the road.
- Local mother-and-baby groups may make you feel less isolated once you have made the initial visit, however difficult it may be to decide to go.
- Try to have some aims to the day, however small.
- Try not to worry about how much there is to do in the house.
- Make yourself eat small appetising meals or milky drinks, and make sure you have easy things to prepare in the house.
- Remember that all women recover from post-natal depression over a period of time. The sooner you ask for help the shorter this period is likely to be.

Returning to work

Many women nowadays have to think about returning to work within a few weeks of their baby being born. If you are going back to work and need to make childcare arrangements, you may wish to talk over the possible choices with your health visitor.

Mothers are often concerned about having to change their baby from feeding from the breast to bottle. In a baby of 7–8 months it is not a worry if the baby refuses milk during the day: three milk feeds – before and after work, and at bedtime – will be enough. Aim to get into this pattern before you actually start back at work.

If a younger baby refuses milk from a bottle or a beaker in the day, he will probably adapt by feeding more from you at night.

This, however, will not help you at an already stressful time. It is therefore advisable to introduce the baby to a bottle or beaker as early as possible. If you are returning to work in the early months you will need to introduce a bottle once breastfeeding is established – when you and the baby both feel confident so that a bottle does not confuse the issue.

TIPS FOR ENCOURAGING BREASTFED BABIES TO DRINK FROM A BOTTLE

- Some babies will take to a bottle with no fuss while others stubbornly refuse it.
- Ask someone who is used to bottlefeeding to try first, as he or she will feel more confident handling the baby and the bottle and this feeling will be transmitted to the baby.
- If you don't know of such a person, it is still better for someone other than the mother (such as Dad) to try as the baby will smell the breastmilk and be far more keen on suckling from Mum.
- Wrap the baby up in a sheet or blanket to feel secure, hold the baby close to you and touch the baby's lips with the teat.
- The baby may become cross if he thinks it is a dummy and not food and may start shaking his head. Loosely hold the teat in the baby's mouth with the teat full of milk but not so that the milk pours into the mouth – drip a little in so that he gets the taste.
- Continue to hold the baby close and rock and talk to him ; once he has calmed down a little he may risk a couple of sucks and realise that it is good.
- Persevere with the bottle despite protests. It might be better for Mum to be out of the house as she will feel awful listening to the struggle. Dad may also feel more confident on his own or with a grandparent there for support.
- Once the baby has taken to the bottle keep him used to it by giving him one every couple of days until you return to work.
- If you aren't having much success, seek advice from your health visitor.
- Parents at Work* is a self-help organisation that provides information on this and other issues.

CHAPTER 5

A GUIDE TO SENSIBLE EATING

FROM the moment of their birth to the day your children leave home, much of your time together will be spent around food and a lot of your own time will be spent in planning, shopping for and cooking their meals. The closeness reached by mother and baby during breast- or bottle-feeding plays a major part in cementing the bond between them. To feed your children well is to respond to a basic instinct, and to see them growing and healthy is an immense satisfaction. Conversely, a lot of worry and tears can result when your baby doesn't feed well, or when your toddler becomes 'picky'. This chapter offers a guide to sensible eating and advice on how to deal with some of the common feeding problems of babies and young children.

Q *What is normal growth?*

A It is useful to know what to expect. The average birth weight for full-term boys or girls is about 3.3kg, but anything between 2.5kg and 4.5kg is normal. Babies should put on about 210gm a week from birth to 3 months, 150gm a week from 3 to 6 months, 90gm a week from 6 to 9 months, and 60gm a week from 9 to 12 months. Your child's weight should be plotted regularly on a centile chart – see pages 58–9. Healthy growth should roughly follow the same line on this chart. A marked deviation upwards (excessive weight gain) or downwards (excessive weight loss) highlights a problem.

Breast-feeding

Breast milk is designed to be best for your newborn baby. The milk you produce in the first few days, called colostrum, contains all the water and nutrients needed for early feeding. While the first flow of mature milk is sweet and watery, the later flow in the same feed is a high-fat, energy-dense milk that contains all the nutrients needed in a sterile, convenient and easily digested form. Breast milk also contains protective antibodies which can help to prevent infections.

Benefits of breast milk

Within breast milk are found enzymes – chemical compounds which promote efficient metabolism. They help achieve optimal absorption; in turn better fat absorption ensures an adequate energy intake for your baby's growth, better calcium uptake, better absorption of many vitamins and minerals and balanced amounts of all fatty acids. Breast milk is also rich in elements from the immune system which fight gastroenteritis and respiratory infections.

Breast-fed babies have less frequent and less severe allergy in those with an allergic family history, and possibly a reduced risk of gastrointestinal problems such as Crohn's or coeliac disease when older.

It may be difficult to establish breast-feeding in some premature or low birth-weight babies and therefore a modified cows'-milk feed may be advised. But often in these cases a mother can express her milk for her baby (see below). The milk is given through a tube which passes down the nostril and the back of the throat to the stomach. It can be supplemented with a breast milk fortifier to provide extra energy, protein, vitamins and minerals. When the baby is strong enough to suck, full breast-feeding can start.

Q *How can I best achieve successful breast-feeding?*

A Successful breast-feeding depends on advance planning. Talk about breast-feeding with your GP, at your ante-natal classes, and with family or friends who have happily breast-fed their own children. Your ante-natal classes will have information about voluntary organisations such as the National Childbirth Trust,★ the Association of Breastfeeding Mothers★ and La Leche League.★

Put your baby to the breast very soon after birth, as a delay in starting is associated with early failure to continue. Remember that it will take a few days to establish the full milk flow. Feed your baby on demand – this may be every two hours in the first few weeks. Don't offer any other fluids, for example, water, or infant formula feeds – there is no need in a well baby. Don't worry if your baby's stools are loose, or a yellow-green colour, as this is normal with breast-feeding.

Don't feel bad if you want to breast-feed but it just doesn't work out. Your baby will grow well on a modified cows'-milk formula.

Q *How can I express breast milk?*

A If you want to breast-feed exclusively but cannot be with your baby for every meal, for example if you are going back to work, or just going out for an evening, you could try using a breast pump to collect your milk, but don't feel bad if you cannot always manage this. Most babies will happily accept a substitute formula feed. Once breast-feeding is well established you can allow yourself some flexibility. You don't have to give up if for some reason you can't breast-feed for a short while – even after a few days without suckling, breast-feeding can be successfully resumed.

Q *Should I give 'top-up' or 'complementary' feeds?*

A A common reason for giving up breast-feeding, often at about six weeks, is the mother's conviction that she is not producing enough milk. She may wish to continue breast-feeding but not feel confident enough to do so. Alternatively, she may think of giving formula feeds as a 'top-up'. However, these complementary feeds remove the stimulus to milk production that results from continuing to offer the breast whenever the baby is hungry. The mother's milk thus becomes relatively less sufficient.

If you are worried that you do not have enough milk, your first response should be to increase the frequency of feeds. Take every opportunity to put your baby to the breast. Your milk flow will increase after a few days. Remember that the more you breast-feed, the more milk you will produce.

Your baby will be weighed and this weight plotted on a centile chart (see above). You will see at a glance if your baby is not getting enough nourishment if the weight line is falling away on the graph. Often your baby will be growing normally and it is just a feeling that you are not producing enough milk. If the weight gain is inadequate your health visitor will discuss with you ways of improving your milk supply, such as checking the correct positioning of your baby at the breast and ensuring you are eating well and taking enough fluids, and advise you on how to get some rest and relaxation. In some circumstances you may be advised to use top-up bottle feeds, but keep breast-feeding as well.

Other common breast-feeding problems

This can be an emotional and tiring time for you, with lots of easy tears. Don't be put off breast-feeding just because of a few early problems. Practical and emotional support from someone outside of the family can help. Ask your midwife or health visitor for advice – she will be supportive and reassuring. Remember that she deals with such problems all the time.

Q *Do I need to eat more when breast-feeding?*

A You will need about an extra 500 calories each day in your own diet before you wean your baby; your protein requirements will also be a little higher. Your health visitor will advise you on how best to realise your own nutritional needs. Don't try to lose weight while breast-feeding as this may decrease the milk volume.

Q *Do I need to avoid any foods while I'm breast-feeding?*

A Alcohol, caffeine and some prescribed drugs can pass into your breast milk. Don't drink too much coffee, tea or fizzy drinks with added caffeine, e.g. colas. Check with your doctor or pharmacist how any drug you are about to take may affect your milk. Cows'-milk protein and other sensitising substances (allergens) can also get into your breast milk and can cause infantile colic or other allergic problems in a sensitive baby (see below). Get advice from a state-registered dietitian in these cases.

Q *How long should I breast-feed for?*

A Babies need to be breast-fed for at least 13 weeks to get the most benefit from your milk. Even if you stop breast-feeding then, the protection gained against bowel and respiratory infection will persist throughout the first year. From six months breast milk on its own cannot supply adequate amounts of iron, copper or zinc and weaning should begin, but many vitamins and minerals will still be more readily absorbed from breast milk. Even small amounts are therefore a useful addition to the weaning diet. If possible, try to continue breast-feeding throughout weaning for the whole of the first year. A period of continued breast-feeding while other foods are introduced is a natural progression for both the baby and you. If you have to stop before one year, substitution with a formula milk is appropriate. After one year of age, whole cows' milk is an adequate drink.

Q *Should I give my breast-fed baby additional vitamins?*

A A deficiency of vitamin K can be associated with easy bleeding and therefore all babies are given a single supplement at birth. Providing your own diet is adequate, babies under six months of age do not require additional vitamins. Between six and twelve months of age, babies who are entirely breast-fed should have supplements of vitamins A, D and C; these are available from your clinic.

Bottle-feeding

If successful breast-feeding has not been established or 'top-up' feeds are required, you can choose one of the nutritionally complete formula feeds available. These feeds are usually based on cows' milk which has been modified to make its nutritional composition very similar to that of breast milk. Formula feeds do not, however, give protection against allergy and infection in the way that breast milk does.

There are four main types of infant formula:

- **pre-term formulae** e.g. Nutriprem (Cow & Gate), Prematil (Milupa), Osterprem (Farley's), SMA Gold LBW (SMA Nutrition)
- **whey-protein-predominant formulae** e.g. Aptamil (Milupa), Premium (Cow & Gate), Farley's First and SMA Gold (SMA Nutrition)
- **casein-protein-predominant formulae** e.g. Cow & Gate Plus, Farley's Second, Milumil (Milupa) and SMA White (SMA Nutrition)
- **follow-on formulae** e.g. Farley's Follow-on Formula, Progress (SMA Nutrition), Step-up (Cow & Gate).

Q *Which formula milk should I choose?*

A Formulae based on whey protein most closely resemble breast milk and are therefore the most commonly chosen feeds for new-born babies. Whey is the watery part of milk which separates out when the milk curdles. At around two or three months of age babies occasionally appear hungry even though they are taking acceptable amounts of formula. In this situation, mothers are often advised to change to one of the formulae based on casein protein (one of the major proteins in cows' milk), commonly thought better at satisfying hunger. Whey- and casein-based milks differ only in the type of their major protein, but have exactly the same nutritional content.

Q *What are pre-term formulae?*

A Premature babies have low nutritional reserves and are considerably smaller than infants that grow to full term in the womb. They have more growing to do and therefore have greater nutritional requirements. Pre-term formulae are higher in energy, protein, sodium, vitamins and minerals than milks designed for full-term babies. Once your infant reaches 2kg a normal formula can be introduced, providing that growth is satisfactory.

Q *What are follow-on formulae?*

A These milks are designed to be used from six months of age. The main difference between standard and follow-on formulae is in the latter's higher iron and protein content. At six months of age, however, most infants will be taking sufficient iron from their weaning diet, so there is no need to change their milk.

If you are weaning your baby on to a vegetarian or vegan diet, or even one that simply avoids red meat, or if your baby dislikes red meat, he or she may be getting less iron than is necessary so a follow-on formula may be useful.

Q *How much milk should I give my baby?*

A The nutritional needs of your baby during the first four months will be met by feeding about 150ml (5fl oz) infant formula for every kilogram of body weight each day.

Newborn baby	510ml (17fl oz)
One month old	630ml (21fl oz)
Two months old	750ml (25fl oz)
Three months old	900ml (30fl oz)
Four months old	960ml (32fl oz)

This gives guidelines only and the amounts will fluctuate on a daily basis. For the first two to three weeks feeds should be given every two to three hours. After this four-hourly feeds or feeding on demand is acceptable. After the introduction of solids at around four months of age the volume of milk needed will gradually decrease. As they approach one year of age most babies will be taking approximately 600ml (20fl oz) of formula a day. If you are worried about the amount of milk that your baby is taking ask your health visitor. Problems are quite often easily sorted out, for instance, a poor milk intake may be due to the type of teat on the bottle.

Q *Should I give my bottle-fed baby additional vitamins?*

A Babies born prematurely are often given a multivitamin supplement, folic acid and iron, usually started in hospital, because of their increased requirements. Providing sufficient infant formula is given (see above) there is no need to give additional vitamins or minerals to a full-term infant. If the amount of formula taken falls below 510ml (17fl oz) during the first year, an additional vitamin supplement containing vitamins A and D must be given. You can obtain this from your doctor or clinic.

Q *When should my baby use a feeder cup?*

A You can start trying to give some of the feeds from a feeder cup from six to nine months of age. Discourage the daytime use of a bottle from one year of age. A feeder cup can be introduced from about six months, to prevent tooth decay and enhance feeding development.

Q *When should I stop using infant formula?*

A Full-fat cows' milk can be introduced at one year of age. The protein and sodium content of cows' milk is too high for your baby before this age and may put stress on the kidneys. If your child's energy intake and growth is good, semi-skimmed milk can be introduced at two years of age. Fully skimmed milk should not be given to children under five years due to its inadequate energy and fat-soluble vitamin content.

Q *What if my baby won't take cows' milk?*

A Cows' milk tastes different to formula or breast milk. If your baby dislikes it you could disguise the taste by mixing it in increasing quantities with formula milk until the taste is accepted. This method is better than using sweetened flavourings.

Q *Should I give my baby additional water or juice?*

A This is not usually necessary during the first four months, unless the weather is exceptionally hot. Once weaning foods have been introduced and providing your baby maintains a good intake of breast or formula milk, you could give him or her additional cooled boiled water or diluted fruit juices. Gradually water or juice will replace one of the milk feeds when solids are taken. Avoid highly sweetened juices (see below). Your baby will need extra water in hot weather or if he or she has a temperature.

Weaning

Aim to introduce solid foods when your baby is between four and six months of age. There are many reasons why this is necessary:

- your baby may still feel hungry after a feed
- breast milk or formula no longer supplies all the nutrients necessary for growth
- the introduction of new textures promotes feeding development and prevents feeding problems in the future
- feeding development is closely linked to speech development, promoting the maturation and co-ordination of the muscles of the tongue and palate.

Q *Which foods should I use?*

A Baby rice mixed either with expressed breast milk or infant formula is usually the first choice. Alternatively, you could use non-wheat cereals, puréed fruits or vegetables. Do not add salt to foods and keep sugar to the minimum required to improve the palatability of sour fruits. From six months of age the variety of foods in the diet, including meat, fish, eggs and all cereals, should be increased.

Q *How much food should I give?*

A Initially, give your baby one to two teaspoonfuls at one feed time per day (usually when he or she is the most hungry). After a week or two, you can introduce solids at a second feed. Between five and six months of age solids are usually taken three times a day – at breakfast, lunch and tea-time feeds. By one year of age your baby will probably be having three meals and two to three snacks a day.

Q *When can I introduce lumpy food?*

A Your baby will be able to experiment with mashed, rather than puréed, food between six and nine months of age. This stage in feeding is necessary for chewing and speech development. Towards one year of age your baby should tolerate chopped food. By this time you should be able to offer him or her a mixed and varied diet.

Q *What about finger foods?*

A Give your baby fingers of toast, rusks, slices of apple and so on between six and nine months of age. It is also important to encourage your baby to play with food, learning how to feed himself or herself. This will undoubtedly result in a great deal of mess, but it is essential! Because of the risk of choking, infants should never be left alone while feeding.

Q *What foods should my baby avoid?*

A The main items are goats' and sheep's milk; certain soft drinks, tea, salt and high-fibre foods.

Goats' or sheep's milk
These milks are sometimes portrayed as less allergy-provoking or more nutritious than cows' milk, but such claims cannot be substantiated by scientific testing. Like unmodified cows' milk, goats' and sheep's milk are low in folic acid, vitamins A and D and iron, and are not safe for infants less than about 12 months old. If you use them for an older infant, take precautions against mineral and vitamin deficiency, and give proper care to their safe preparation – they must be pasteurised or boiled.

Sugar

Sugar damages children's teeth (see Chapter 7). Keep intake to a minimum.

- Try to avoid foods that contain concentrated fruit juices (see page 130), sucrose and glucose such as baby fruit juices, syrup-based drinks and excessive cakes or sweets.
- Don't dip a dummy in a sweet drink.
- Don't use honey as a sweetener.
- Don't give sweetened, or naturally sweet, drinks from a bottle – repeatedly bathing the teeth in a sweet solution increases the risk of potential decay.
- Try to encourage a feeder cup rather than a bottle, the reason being that a feeder cup has a shorter contact time between the teeth and the potentially damaging feeds. (Other fruit juices should be diluted.)

Certain drinks

Don't offer other 'soft drinks' like colas that can contain caffeine or other stimulants. 'Diet' soft drinks may result in too high an intake of artificial sweeteners, and fizzy drinks are not suitable for weaning. Tea is not suitable as a main drink for young children, as it can reduce the absorption of iron and other minerals. Sugar added to tea is also a risk to dental health.

Salt

Never add salt to food as it can overload the kidneys of a young child.

High-fibre foods

An excessive intake of high-fibre foods should be avoided, especially in early infancy. High-fibre foods are difficult to digest and are low in energy, which could result in an inadequate energy intake and poor growth. However, some infants have problems with constipation and wholewheat cereals (not bran), fruits and vegetables are helpful in preventing this.

Early eating problems

Q *My baby won't feed – what can I do?*

A Poor feeding is usually easily dealt with. Check the following: milk flow, that the teat is not too small or too large, and that the milk is not too hot; does your baby need 'winding' during the feed?; is the nose blocked? is he comfortable at the breast? are you allowing sufficient time for feeding? Remember that a sudden reluctance to feed may be a sign of general illness. If your baby is feverish, lethargic, or in any other way 'not himself', contact your doctor.

Q *My baby has colic – what should I do?*

A Some babies experience abdominal pain after feeding. This often just disappears after three months, the so-called 'three-month colic'. Much of this is probably because the newborn gut is 'acclimatising' to life outside the womb. It may cause distress but does not lead to any harm, and settles easily without any medical intervention. Colic can, however, be an important sign of intolerance to cows'-milk protein passing through breast milk. This should be considered if any of these features apply:

- a family history of food allergy
- a hungry baby who feeds eagerly but stops soon
- the baby cries as if in pain
- the baby draws up the legs after a short feed
- general irritability
- vomiting and frequent loose stools
- poor weight gain
- eczema, or a skin rash that comes on with feeding or after skin contact with milk.

Remember that food allergy is not always the cause of these symptoms and you should consult your doctor. The use of gripe-water or any other 'over-the-counter' remedies is unlikely to help. Some parents have found that cranial osteopathy or homeopathy may give relief.

Q *What should I do if my baby's colic is due to cows'-milk allergy?*

A See 'food allergy' below.

Q *My baby keeps vomiting – what should I do?*

A Most babies bring back a small amount of milk after some feeds. This 'posseting' is of no significance. A few babies will have gastro-oesophageal reflux (reflux, for short). This is characterised by effortless vomiting, which may continue between feeds. It is caused by an immaturity of the stomach muscles and valves, so the milk is simply regurgitated. Your GP may diagnose reflux on the basis of the symptoms described by you, but may decide to confirm it by x-ray. Bottle-fed babies with reflux will often respond to a milk thickener which your doctor can prescribe. Early weaning to a more solid diet can help. This must be supervised by your doctor or health visitor. Never add solids to bottles for these reasons:

- unless solids are given by the normal routes a baby will not learn to use a spoon
- solids in bottles will fill up a baby too much, so that he or she is not hungry enough to experiment with solids by the normal route
- solids in bottles can lead to sucking difficulties as the milk will be rendered too thick.

If the reflux is severe your GP may suggest a medicine which stimulates the gut muscles to push the feed down through the stomach. It is very rare for reflux to cause any serious problem, and it usually settles spontaneously in the first year. Rarely, vomiting is a sign of a more severe disorder. If it is bile-stained or very forceful contact your doctor immediately. Remember also that vomiting can be the first sign of an illness in your baby or young child. The source of the problem may not lie in the tummy – it could be an ear or waterworks infection.

Later problems

Q *My child won't eat – what can I do?*

A The 'terrible 2-year-old' with highly individual food tastes and eating patterns is very common. Any toddler may frustrate his or her parents by refusing food. You should look on this as a variation on normal behaviour, perhaps as a way of getting more attention. It shows that your child is learning to manipulate people and social situations. Though you may be driven to despair, especially if you have other young children, remember that it is a temporary condition. It will not cause any harm and you can deal with it.

GOOD MEALS GUIDE

- Have regular mealtimes.
- Try to eat as a family – your child will enjoy eating with you.
- Ensure that all members of the family (including grandparents) apply a consistent approach to eating habits.
- Encourage your child by praising all good eating behaviour, and ignoring food refusal as much as possible.
- Make meals fun with brightly coloured plates and attractively prepared food.
- Limit in-between snacking.
- Seek advice if you are making no progress or losing your patience, or if your child is not gaining weight, or if the diet is so faddy that you are worried about dietary deficiency.
- Don't let the meal go on and on – a good rule is to limit mealtimes to 30 minutes.
- Don't offer an alternative meal.
- Don't criticise your child.
- Never force your child to eat.

Loss of appetite, rather than difficult eating habits, may reflect some emotional upset or be a general sign of ill health. If you have any such concerns consult your doctor.

Q *My child is overweight – what should I do?*

A Don't worry if your baby or toddler seems fat. Most infants will lose weight as they become more mobile and active. Most overweight children will 'grow into' their weight during their teenage years. If your child is really overweight, often a simple avoidance, or reduced intake, of chocolate, biscuits, crisps and so on will be all that is needed. Don't start any fashionable diets and have realistic objectives. Any weight loss should be gradual; alternatively, it may be acceptable to maintain the current weight until weight and height are appropriate. At this time regular, but not too frequent, visits to your doctor can be an important source of encouragement for your child. Acute slimming can be dangerous and in the susceptible child, even at around 10 years of age, can precipitate anorexia nervosa.

Don't make a family issue of it or weigh your child every day. If you feel that no progress is being made, or that your child's weight is a cause of misery or family tensions, discuss your worries with your doctor, who may feel that referral for a specialist paediatric opinion is needed.

Avoidance of dietary deficiencies

For full-term babies breast or formula milks are nutritionally complete for the first six months of life. After this age infants and children who eat a normal and varied diet are not at risk of dietary deficiency. Older children with little exposure to sunlight may need extra vitamin D and those who develop 'faddy' eating habits may benefit from added vitamins or minerals.

The child's diet should be assessed by a paediatric dietitian and supplemented only with proper supervision. Remember, excessive doses of some vitamins, for example vitamin A, can damage the liver.

Food allergy

Although cows' milk is the most frequently implicated food, intolerance to soya, egg and wheat is also relatively common. More or less any food is capable of causing a reaction.

High-risk babies
Some babies may be at an increased risk of developing symptoms. This can be identified by a strong family history of allergic-based disorders such as asthma, eczema, allergic runny nose, and skin rashes like nettle sting. If you think your baby is at an increased risk discuss this with your doctor and midwife. If you are going to breast-feed and the risk is thought to be high enough, you may be asked to avoid the major food allergens in your own diet just before your baby is born, and while breast-feeding.

If you plan to bottle-feed your baby, there may be some benefit in using a very low-allergy formula – one can be prescribed by your doctor. Breast-feeding or the use of the specialised formula should continue until your baby is at least 12 months old. Although you should introduce solids at the normal age of four to six months, delay the introduction of foods known to provoke allergies, such as cows' milk, soya, wheat and eggs.

If you notice a reaction following the introduction of any food make sure you avoid it. The decision to undertake these allergy prevention treatments should be made by careful assessment of the baby in question, with specialist advice from a paediatrician and dietitian to ensure both the nutritional adequacy of your own and your baby's diet, and complete avoidance of the suspect food.

Allergy prevention for other babies

The most beneficial thing you can do is to breast-feed your baby. You can further reduce the possibility of food allergy by excluding from the diet until six months of age, foods which may provoke an allergy such as egg and wheat. Gluten-free weaning cereals like rice or maize, given until six months, will help to minimise the risk of coeliac disease (see page 161), an allergic response to gluten that damages the small intestine and interferes with food absorption.

Treatment of known cows'-milk allergy

If you are breast-feeding it may be necessary to exclude cows' milk and its products from your own diet, as small amounts will pass into your breast milk. Substitute cows' milk with other types of milk. Bottle-fed infants will usually be given a modified soya-based infant formula. However, a proportion of infants with cows' milk intolerance will go on to develop a secondary soya intolerance, and if so a very low-allergenic formula milk may be required. Your doctor will prescribe these milks.

Normal unmodified soya milk is not nutritionally complete for babies and should not be used before one year of age. If cows'-milk intolerance is your baby's problem you will see an immediate and dramatic improvement after changing to one of the prescribed milks.

Q *Will my baby always be intolerant to the food?*

A No. By the age of one year most infants have grown out of their problems. Your doctor or dietitian will advise you how to check this by introducing a small amount of the food into your baby's diet.

Q *Can food intolerance occur in later childhood?*

A Yes. A number of conditions, such as failure to thrive, diarrhoea, asthma, eczema, migraine and behavioural problems, can be caused or aggravated by food intolerance. The food responsible for the allergy may be obvious and easy to avoid, or much more difficult to pinpoint. In this case a closely supervised, complex food exclusion diet may be required. Your GP or dietitian should ensure that your child's diet is nutritionally adequate and give you advice on food re-introduction (food challenges).

Q *Are reactions with food challenges ever dangerous?*

A Very occasionally there can be a very severe reaction called 'anaphylaxis' (see page 43). This can occur at any age and is most commonly caused by peanuts or eggs. The intolerance in these children is usually life-long and food avoidance must be very strict.

Q *Can I have my child tested for food allergies?*

A Blood tests are not 100 per cent reliable in identifying allergies, and are best used as a guide in determining whether specific food allergies are likely or not. Before manipulating a child's diet, your GP or dietitian would want to view the whole clinical picture. There are many alternative allergy-testing clinics using techniques for diagnosis that have not been scientifically proven. Many of these tests are expensive and can be difficult to justify.

Vegetarian diets

Q *Can I feed my baby a vegetarian diet?*

A Yes. Vegetarian foods can be introduced in the normal way. If you are vegetarian and are breast-feeding your baby you must ensure that your own vitamin D, calcium and iron intake is adequate.

Q *Do vegetarian foods provide all the nutrients required by my baby?*

A Providing your baby is taking an adequate amount of infant formula or breast milk you can be confident that his or her diet is nutritionally complete. In the older child iron is the only nutrient which may be low, as red meat is its main source. The inclusion of eggs, peas, beans and lentils in the diet from six months will help to ensure an adequate iron intake. Foods containing vitamin C, such as oranges and tomatoes, will enhance the absorption of iron from these sources.

For young infants it is best to remove the skin from peas and beans after cooking to prevent excessive bulk in the diet. The use of a follow-on formula in babies over six months will also help to improve their iron intake. As your child gets older the diet will be nutritionally adequate providing you offer a good variety of milk products, eggs, peas, beans, lentils and nuts (very finely ground to avoid the risk of choking) each day, alongside vegetables, fruit and cereals. Children with a history of food allergy should avoid nuts.

Q *Is a vegan diet suitable for my child?*

A A vegan diet, which excludes meat, fish, eggs and animal milks, can be inadequate in energy, vitamin and mineral content. If you want your baby to follow this type of diet it is of paramount importance that you plan carefully, take expert dietetic advice, and monitor the growth of the child. Breast milk or a suitable nutritionally complete vegan infant formula must be given to all infants. You will need to acquire a detailed knowledge of acceptable foods rich in vitamins and minerals. Even with this knowledge, however, additional vitamin and mineral supplementation may be required.

Eating for the future

Many parents ask whether, and if so, when, low-fat, low-sugar and high-fibre healthy eating principles should be applied to the diets of children. The nutritional requirements in this age group are very different from those of adults. An infant requires a much higher daily energy intake per kilogram of body weight. Fat and refined carbohydrate are very concentrated forms of energy and are therefore important to infants and children. Fifty per cent of the energy in breast and formula milk comes from fat. These milks also have a high proportion of simple sugars and are low in fibre. For these reasons if solids which are predominantly low in fat and high in fibre are introduced the resulting diet will be low in energy and poor growth may result. 'Healthy diet' principles do not generally apply to children under two years of age. However, fruits, vegetables and wholegrain cereals are recommended within a balanced diet. After two years of age, you can offer semi-skimmed milk and gently cut down on fat intake as well as increasing fibre, providing the diet remains nutritionally adequate.

Fully skimmed milk should not be introduced before five years of age. At this stage parents should start to encourage children to eat a more 'healthy diet'. It is important to remember, however, that the energy requirements always need to be high to support the growth of children and that over-zealous application of adult healthy eating principles (the so-called 'muesli belt syndrome') may result in irreversible growth failure.

CHAPTER 6

BEHAVIOURAL AND EMOTIONAL PROBLEMS

IT is easy to watch the dramatic physical development of your child and forget that huge emotional and behavioural changes are happening at the same time. Babies, virtually from the start, are unique in their temperaments, sleeping patterns and what can make them laugh or cry.

It may be hard to think of children developing emotional or even psychiatric problems but some do: it is estimated that between 10 and 20 per cent of children will at some point develop a problem that will affect their mental health. Though many of these problems – such as feeling anxious or miserable – would not be considered serious, to the affected child they are a problem.

Who is at risk?

As with adults who develop psychological problems, it is rare to be able to pinpoint one particular cause, even if to do so might be tempting. In reality it is a lot more complicated. Some factors are:

- low intelligence, making it harder for children to react to stressful or adverse circumstances
- chronic physical ill health, particularly when a child suffers chronic pain or is in hospital for a prolonged stay
- developmental delay: a poor ability to communicate may put the child at risk of developing emotional problems
- poor family discipline
- grief at the death of a parent, brother or sister or other close relative

- physical, sexual or emotional abuse
- poor parental health, particularly if the parent suffers from a psychiatric illness such as depression
- the cultural background – this will have an important role in formulating a child's emotional reactions.

Tackling an emotional or behavioural problem

If you seek professional help for such a problem you might see a teacher or a health professional such as your GP or health visitor. Talking it through may in itself help both you and your child by putting the problem into perspective. The professional may, however, suggest that your child should be assessed by others.

The GP may already have held informal discussions with (and possibly obtained some reports from) the teacher, the school nurse or the health visitor. Sometimes the GP may refer a patient to a child and adolescent psychiatrist.

Whoever is carrying out the assessment will obtain a detailed picture from you, the parents, to clarify the exact nature of the problem. At the same time the therapist will observe your reactions and will watch how the child responds to you. If the GP or the usual health visitor is involved he or she is likely to have the advantage of already knowing your family and any problems. A child psychiatrist will not usually have prior information but should have some background details from the GP on the referral letter. A child who is old enough may be interviewed on his or her own. The therapist has to take into account the age of the child when assessing appropriate behaviour as well as the social and cultural background. It may well be that more than one session is required to build up a proper picture.

Behavioural and emotional problems in infants and younger children

All infants and their parents have to get over the various hurdles of establishing **sleep** routines, dealing with **crying** and **temper tantrums** and learning **bladder and bowel control**. For more information on all these subjects and some of those that follow, see Chapter 4.

Delayed development

Poor stimulation of a baby or a child may significantly limit and impair a child's emotional and behavioural development. A good example is that of a child left alone for hours on end with no toys or stimulation: the child can become withdrawn and uninterested in anything. Sometimes this emotional deprivation affects a child's general well-being and the term 'failure to thrive' may be used. Such babies or children are often underweight in comparison with their peers.

Failure to thrive is a non-specific diagnosis that can cover a multitude of disorders and situations; some of them will have a physical basis. For example, coeliac disease and cystic fibrosis are conditions which may cause failure to thrive. Emotionally deprived babies may initially seem to be failing to thrive: when they are admitted to hospital, fed regularly and given proper stimulation, they start thriving again. If discharged back into the old situation they slip back into the previous state. Once the problem is recognised and families receive the treatment and help that they need, the majority of these children will ultimately develop normally.

Speech problems

Not surprisingly parents will become anxious if their child is slow to speak, particularly when their peers are starting to utter their first words. It's important to realise that just like many of the milestones in a child's development, there is a huge variation of what can be defined as normal. Often the first recognisable word is detected at about ten months, but every child is different, and even at 13 months one in ten children still cannot form a word that is comprehensible. If your child falls into this category there are two questions you can ask yourself:

- Is my child developing normally otherwise?
- Can my child hear?

The latter question is crucial – a deaf child should receive immediate medical attention and assessment. If the child cannot hear there is little chance that proper speech will develop. Hearing develops very early – by about two months your baby should smile if you speak directly to him. By about three months he should turn when he hears a familiar voice and from five months onwards he should be able to localise the source of a sound accurately.

Stammering

Stammering is common and about 1 in 20 children under the age of five will have fluency problems while learning to talk. Many children will grow out of it but some don't. If a child has fluency problems with speech for more than six months there may be grounds for anxiety. An early referral for speech and language therapy may be appropriate – discuss this with your health visitor or GP. Certainly, children who start stammering at school should be promptly referred for specialist help. Children with a family history of stammering are at particular risk and need careful observation.

A new baby in the family

Two children in a family can have more than double the effect of just one child. This is particularly true if there is only a small age gap between the two. Although the parents may have experience of bringing up children, having to cope with the change can be difficult. The whole family has to adjust but it is the older child or children who may encounter the biggest difficulties. How can you ease the change?

- If at all possible, discuss with the older child or children the idea of a new baby coming into the family. Use picture books and stories or draw examples from friends, families or neighbours.
- There may be changes such as a new room or new sleeping arrangements. Perhaps the older child may have to vacate the cot. All these should be introduced slowly – don't do them all at once. If at all possible try to have any changes in place before the new arrival.
- Try to keep to roughly the same routines and activities before and after the birth.
- Don't expect the older child to share the same enthusiasm for the new arrival as everyone else. In fact, you may notice a return to more baby-like behaviour, such as wanting a bottle.

- If friends are bringing a present for the new baby ask if they might bring a small gift for the older child too.
- Be patient and tolerant – not easy, but who said being a parent was easy?

Although there may initially be some jealousy at a new arrival, over a period of time new babies will be incorporated as part of their close circle. In fact, it is thought that babies may become attached to their brothers and sisters within the first year of life. As these babies get older they will become more confident and adventurous when a big brother or sister is in the vicinity.

The dyslexic child

There is tremendous confusion over what exactly constitutes dyslexia. The word is derived from the Greek and means 'difficulty with words'. Another term for dyslexia is 'specific learning disability', which conveys the fact that the problems are specific rather than global.

Dyslexia boils down to a problem in learning to read or spell in a child who is otherwise developing normally. In particular, there may be no intellectual impairment, so dyslexic children may appear intelligent in normal conversation but when it comes to written work or reading they are obviously struggling; they may also have problems with numeracy and music. Other difficulties associated with dyslexia include clumsiness and a poor ability to concentrate.

The true cause of the condition essentially remains unknown. It is thought that abnormalities in specific areas of the brain, particularly those areas that deal with language and speech, are responsible. It is possible that the complex internal wiring of the brain may be disturbed – research into this continues. With modern imaging technology, previously inaccessible areas are now being visualised; this may give some clue as to the causes of dyslexia.

It is well recognised that dyslexia can run in families, so it is tempting to say that it has a genetic link but, again, this has not been proven. Dyslexia is much more common than people realise, with 4 per cent of the population significantly affected. Put another way, at least one child in every class is likely to be affected.

In many children dyslexia is not identified until late on at nursery school or even at infant school, when they start to use letters and numbers on a regular basis. A family history of dyslexia may act as a warning sign but sometimes no other member of the family is affected.

Some children can be smart enough to disguise their disabilities and will simply be classed as under-achievers at school, while others may appear just to be clumsy in eye and hand co-ordination.

The pre-school child
Look for the following in a pre-school child:

- jumbled and confused words or mixed-up phrases
- clumsiness – falls a great deal or is poor at dressing himself or herself
- speech delay
- poor concentration.

This kind of behaviour can be difficult to differentiate from a normally developing child so don't be unduly worried. But where the problems are persistent and severe or a number of them seem to apply, dyslexia should be considered.

The schoolchild
The problems start to become more obvious when a child is having difficulty in reading and writing. He may have difficulty in telling left from right and may regularly and wrongly reverse digits and letters. A dyslexic child may also be clumsy and will take longer than his peers to do written work. This slow progress in reading and writing will contrast with other markers of intelligence – in fact, many dyslexic children prove on further testing to be of above average intelligence. As they grow older their ability to keep up with their non-dyslexic peers becomes harder. This can lead to frustration, poor self-esteem and even behavioural problems. In a world where the written word is a fundamental linchpin of communication, dyslexia can be a major disability.

Tackling the problem of dyslexia
The child with delayed speech development and a poor vocabulary should be fully assessed, particularly in terms of hearing and general development. The diagnosis of dyslexia can often be confirmed or suggested by a psychologist able to estimate the degree

of reading difficulty. The psychologist would also gauge whether other problems such as low intelligence or poor schooling are causing the reading difficulties. An assessment can be arranged through the school.

When a decision is made that a child has dyslexia or 'specific learning disability', it may come as a shock to the family. Whatever word is used, it is essential for the child to understand that he has a specific disability. Equally important is the fact that both teachers and parents understand the nature of the disability. Once this is understood, progress in overcoming the child's learning difficulties will be made.

As parents you need to provide your child with support and encourage him in activities in which he can succeed. Take into account the fact that he will have to work much harder than his peers and yet will not make as much progress. In the process he can find this tiring as well as demoralising, so try to keep up his morale.

In addition, parents and teachers should maintain good lines of communication with each other about his progress. The child who is identified early and receives appropriate teaching and support should fare well and maximise his potential. The problem is identifying dyslexic children early. Though a child may not grow out of it, there are methods which can minimise its effects.

The autistic child

Few conditions are as misunderstood as autism. Many people who saw the film *Rain Man* erroneously assume that all autistic people are gifted. In fact, about half of all autistic people will be classified as having a severe learning disability – that is, an IQ of less than 50 – while only a quarter are in the normal range.

Although autism can be associated with other forms of mental handicap, it is classified as a developmental disorder which can cause an abnormality of social interaction, communication and imagination. In a way, an autistic child is cut off from the outside world. Autism is not common and estimates of its prevalence vary but a reasonable estimate is that approximately 1 child in 2,500 is affected. However, some children may exhibit some 'milder' forms of autism, making the incomplete version much commoner, affecting perhaps 1 in every 500 children. In common with other developmental disorders, boys are at much greater risk of developing this disorder.

Children with autistic tendencies may display any of the following symptoms:

- bizarre and difficult-to-control behaviour
- will not play with other children
- irrational fears and obsessional rituals
- poor speech; sometimes complete absence of speech
- repetition of words with no concept of meaning
- about one-third of autistic children will develop epilepsy by adolescence.

Autism is neither a psychiatric illness nor a juvenile form of schizophrenia; nor is it a disorder of the middle class. Like many developmental disorders the features unfold as the child grows and develops. Since poor communication is the main handicap, the signs will start to show at around 18 months but will become more noticeable by the age of three. Diagnosis can be painfully slow and it may take several years before the penny drops. Treatment involves specialised advice, full support to the family and a great deal of patience.

Disruption to their rigid routines will cause severe upset to autistic children, particularly to those with obsessional tendencies. With patience, routines can slowly be changed; helping children to predict change can also be useful. You could also try non-verbal means of communication such as a drawing or pictures to try to bring about a gentle change in their routines.

Other coping strategies:

- As with other children, rules must be clear and consistent.
- Bizarre behaviour may be the only way that the autistic child can communicate with other people. Sometimes you as carers have to accept this.
- Be patient.
- Encourage your child to develop new skills.

The hyperactive child

Hyperactivity is a word that is banded about rather loosely, so it is important to define the problem more precisely. A hyperactive child is one who is over-active and displays significant inattention and impulsiveness. The result is chaotic and disorganised behaviour which if severe enough may adversely affect normal development. This anti-social conduct can lead to problems in learning and can put considerable strain on both the family and the school. Sometimes the term 'attention deficit disorder' is used as an alternative to 'hyperactivity' at the severe end of the spectrum.

Severe hyperactivity is also called hyperkinetic disorder; in the UK, the diagnosis will be made only when all three main features – impulsiveness, over-activity and inattention – are present. In addition, their presence should be consistent at school and at home. About 0.5 per cent of children can fit within this strict diagnostic definition.

To confuse matters some people use different standards to reach a definition of a hyperactive child. For example, in the United States the criteria needed to make a diagnosis are less stringent. As a result the incidence of the hyperactive disorder is much more common there than in the UK. However, this difference may also partially reflect a degree of under-diagnosis in the UK.

Like many developmental disorders, it is much more common in boys than girls – in this case by a factor of four. No specific cause has been found but numerous reasons may be responsible. Studies in twins have suggested that hereditary factors play a significant role.

The features of impulsiveness, over-activity and inattention have to be placed in the context of the development of the child. For example, it is hard to pin a diagnosis of hyperactivity on a child who has not yet started school. After all, at the pre-school stage, the range of normal activity and attention span varies enormously. The diagnosis of hyperactivity or any of its variants should be made by an expert in the field, such as a child psychiatrist.

As the child grows up, anti-social behaviour may affect school performance and relationships. Although most children will eventually grow out of it or respond to treatment, some will have long-term difficulties that will persist into adult life.

Tackling the problem of hyperactivity
Parents and the immediate family and friends should acquire a good understanding of the condition. One strategy is to reward children for achieving specific goals such as prolonged periods of good conduct. Also, it's sensible to decrease stimulation, such as

117

allowing them to watch television rather than run around, but providing outlets for bursts of physical activity. Extra help may be needed in the classroom and again the focus should be on helping the child to develop a good attention span. Obviously, this requires the full co-operation of the educational authorities and the teachers.

Within conventional medicine, it is unusual to consider drug therapy or even dietary changes to tackle a child's psychological problem, but most experts agree that such a treatment is a possibility for hyperactivity, and that drug therapy should be initiated if the situation is severe or if a major family or school crisis is imminent.

The drugs used include dexamphetamine, methylphenidate and pemoline, which are all brain stimulants. It may seem paradoxical that stimulants are used to treat a condition in which children are already over-stimulated, but scientific trials have shown them to be effective. The best results of drug treatment are in the 5-10 age group. Side effects include an initial difficulty in getting to sleep, a reduction of appetite and, not surprisingly, a lowering of the general mood. The child's height and weight should be regularly recorded because these drugs can affect growth, though the effects tend to be mild and the final adult height and weight are not usually affected.

Initially, a 4-8-week period of drug treatment will be tried to see if there is a significant improvement. Those children who respond well may need regular treatment, sometimes for several years. Every so often, perhaps once a year, the treatment should be stopped and the need for further treatment assessed, depending on the patterns of behaviour observed in the drug-free periods.

A change in eating habits may produce some benefit for some children. In particular, food additives have taken the blame for hyperactivity and there may be some evidence to back this up. However, special additive-free diets are hard to follow and there may be a risk of causing a nutritional deficiency, so if you are convinced that a certain food is causing your child to have behavioural problems seek advice from a dietitian via your GP.

Behavioural and emotional problems in schoolchildren

Children frequently express worries and anxieties that are very similar to those of adults, although the content of these fears will obviously reflect the child's age, intelligence and education. Normal children with normal fears will gradually be able to develop coping strategies, but if the anxiety becomes disproportionate and out of context, it will have a detrimental effect on the child's behaviour. In some cases certain events such as bereavement or a break-up of the family may contribute to the overall problem.

You will need to listen and talk with your child a great deal and acquire an understanding of the reasons for his anxieties. You need to help your child face up to the situations that he finds anxiety-provoking. For instance, if he is refusing to attend school (see below), encourage rather than bully him to return to school. If this approach does not work, you may need to enlist expert help in the form of a psychologist or a child psychiatrist.

True clinical depression is rare in a child who has yet to arrive at puberty; if this is genuinely thought to be the problem the child should be assessed by a child psychiatrist. In the adolescent, the incidence of depression starts to climb; symptoms to look out for include a lowered mood, excessive tiredness and a withdrawal from friends. In addition, there may a curbing of the appetite, and possible anti-social behaviour.

Anti-social behaviour

Some children – often older ones – display unacceptable behaviour, such as aggressive tendencies, streaks of cruelty or episodes of destructiveness. In addition, such children may also steal, lie or stay out of the house beyond an acceptable time. The tolerance of such behaviour will depend on various factors such as what the family and local community expects and the degree of general family discipline. Some people may dismiss it as high spirits while others will view it as a serious anti-social problem.

It is thought that conduct disorders of this nature are present in roughly 50 per cent of schoolchildren with psychiatric problems and follow the usual pattern of being more common in boys than girls. They are also more common in children from broken homes and dysfunctional families. Some of these children will display a strong temperament from a young age. In severe cases a child psychiatrist may get involved. Treatment will be based on:

- looking at family relationships; this obviously requires the co-operation of the whole family.
- teaching the child and the parents coping strategies to curb the abnormal behaviour.
- getting the school involved (and if necessary social workers).

Unfortunately, many of these children will carry their behaviour patterns with them into adulthood. They can develop problems with relationships, employment and even fall foul of the law.

School refusal and truancy

It is not uncommon for a child to refuse to attend school. At the point of leaving home, a child may have a tantrum, burst into tears and even complain of having a headache or feeling sick.

Truancy is different from school refusal in that often no one knows the whereabouts of a truanting child. Truancy is often associated with a conduct disorder while school refusal is a reflection of an emotional disorder.

Tackling reluctance to attend school

It is important to explore the child's fears and anxieties to get to the bottom of the problem. Sometimes the cause is obvious – perhaps there is bullying at school, a new teacher, difficulties with school work or the child has been involved in a previously undisclosed event in the playground or classroom. Don't forget that a domestic upset or illness may be the culprit.

It is essential to listen and talk to the child. You as parents are in the best position to do this and at the early stages no one else need be involved. If the problem is found to be at the school then obviously you should seek the help of the teaching staff. Occasionally, a change of school may be the answer, but be careful as the school refusal may be repeated at the new school. If a domestic problem is the cause, that should be addressed but efforts should still be made to get the child to attend school. If all else fails the child may benefit from seeing a psychologist specialising in this area.

The best results are obtained when the child returns to school quickly. The longer the absence, the harder it is to solve the problem.

Eating disorders

Eating disorders are rare but not unknown in young children; they tend to be found more commonly in adolescent girls.

There is no one cause of **anorexia nervosa**. The onset is usually insidious and the sufferer will often deny that she has a problem with her eating. She may express a fear of becoming fat and will become obsessed with her shape and body image. As a result she will markedly reduce her food intake, leading to a significant and sometimes extreme weight loss, even emaciation. She may well remain very interested in food and associated topics despite the fact that she will go to great lengths to avoid eating.

Bulimia nervosa is an allied condition in which body weight may actually be maintained. However, the girl may indulge in episodes of binge-eating, and then possibly make herself vomit. She may also abuse laxatives to counteract the binge-eating.

How to tackle eating disorders

The treatment for both conditions is difficult and should be taken very seriously. In a crisis, particularly one brought about by anorexia nervosa, a general medical team may need to deal with any severe medical problems, such as those affecting the metabolism, with the girl as an in-patient. The long-term psychological care should be left to a specialist team which may include specially trained nurses, dietitians, psychologists and occupational therapists as well as a specialist psychiatrist.

Child neglect and abuse

A child may be harmed both physically and emotionally by his parents or carers. They may display aggression towards the child, or ignore his emotional needs. Physical neglect in an extreme case will result in an undernourished, dirty, unkempt child. Very active rashes may spring up at sites where dirt collects – in the nappy area, for example.

Sexual abuse

Sexual abuse of children appears to be on the increase, possibly due to the fact that it is being recognised and acknowledged more frequently. More often than not, the abuser turns out to be either a member of the family or someone well known to the family. Sometimes there may be signs suggestive of sexual abuse, such as vaginal discharge, a sore bottom, disturbed behaviour and even playing that involves the mimicking of sexual acts.

If you suspect that your child may be being sexually abused, try not to panic. Consider asking your GP for advice first, though doctors have an ethical duty to report cases where they are suspicious of such abuse. It is important to obtain the full story before it is coloured by repeated and perhaps leading questioning.

Non-accidental injury

Some parents or guardians sometimes physically abuse children in their care. Physical abuse is called non-accidental injury (NAI) and can occur when parents are at their wits' end with the demands of the child. However, it can also occur when inadequate parents cannot control their own tempers or may be suffering from a mental illness.

Sometimes NAI can be the result of pre-meditated cruelty by the parents. A wide range of injuries can be seen, commonly fingertip bruising on the chest and tummy: these gripping injuries are the result of forceful and excessive handling. Shaking the head vigorously can cause the tearing of veins inside the head, resulting in the formation of blood clots. This in turn can cause excess pressure within the skull and lead to brain damage. Other injuries associated with NAI include bite marks, cigarette burns and bone fractures.

Anyone who suspects an NAI (health professional, social worker, police officer, and so on) should ensure that the child is removed to a safe haven, possibly a hospital. Many children are allowed to return home – but under supervision, usually from the social services. If the child is thought to be at recurrent risk he or she may need to be taken away and placed in the care of others.

All children attract their fair share of bruises and bashes by the very nature of their behaviour and relatively poor co-ordination. Furthermore, bleeding disorders and bones that break easily – brittle bones – can masquerade as non-accidental injury, so it is essential that the team examining a child suspected of suffering an NAI should make every effort to exclude these conditions and consider all other possibilities.

CHAPTER 7

CARE OF YOUR CHILD'S TEETH

CARING for teeth from a very early age is essential to avoid dental problems later in life. This is particularly so because the main dental diseases – tooth decay (caries) and gum disease (periodontal disease) – are largely preventable.

Children's teeth develop in two stages. The first set, also called primary dentition or milk teeth, which number 20, start developing in the jaws long before the baby is born and usually come through into the mouth between the ages of 6 and 30 months. Most of the second set, called permanent dentition or adult teeth, come through between 6 and 13 years of age. Four more teeth – the wisdom teeth – may (or may never) appear after the age of 17, bringing the full complement of permanent teeth to 32.

Tooth decay

The main worry for most parents is that their child's teeth may decay. Tooth decay is caused by a live film of bacteria on the teeth (plaque) that turns sugar from food into acid. This acid dissolves the hard outer layer of enamel of the tooth and a hole (or cavity) develops. If the cavity gets deep enough into the tooth, it will become infected and turn into an abscess, which can be very painful.

A huge amount can now be done to prevent caries from occurring in the first place. The best approach is a three-fold attack on the main causes: plaque, sugar and vulnerable tooth enamel.

Beating plaque

Plaque builds up constantly on teeth and needs to be thoroughly brushed off twice a day. It is much easier for a child to acquire good mouth-keeping habits as soon as the teeth appear rather than later on in life. Try to make it fun. If your child insists on brushing his or her own teeth make sure that an adult gets to do them as well. Make this the last thing the child does at night, after the final meal and drink.

Use a small brush with a pea-sized blob of children's toothpaste and give the teeth a good scrub. Be methodical so that all the surfaces of all the teeth, including the biting surfaces, get cleaned. With small children the easiest way of doing this is to cradle their heads and lean over them, or to get them to lie back on your lap or even on the bathroom floor. It can sometimes be a struggle and you may end up with toothpaste everywhere but on the teeth, but perseverance usually wins. It does get easier with time.

Disclosing tablets

Children do not have the dexterity to clean their teeth properly until they are quite old – say, 10 or 11. They can check on how effective their brushing is by using disclosing tablets. When these harmless tablets, available from pharmacies, are chewed or sucked any plaque left after brushing is stained a bright colour so that it can be easily seen and brushed off.

Floss

Older children can use dental floss to clean in between the teeth where the bristles of a brush cannot reach. Younger children can have their teeth flossed for them – flossing is a great habit to encourage from an early age.

Fissure sealant

Cavities often start in tiny cracks and crevices in the biting surfaces – the pits and fissures – of the back teeth, where plaque readily collects. Tiny cracks can be sealed by a dentist using a fissure sealant, a plastic coating painted on to the teeth that flows into fissures, where it is set rock hard by the use of a special light. The process is painless and is tremendously effective in preventing cavities in the teeth (usually the back permanent teeth). The sealant lasts for many years and can always be reapplied if it chips or comes off.

Reducing sugar

Sugar damages the state of a child's teeth. Sugar is obvious in foods such as sweets but less obvious as a major ingredient in a huge number of other foods. Manufacturers often use other names, such as dextrose and sucrose, in the list of ingredients to hide the presence of what is basically sugar.

As far as dental health is concerned it is not how much sugar the child takes in that matters but the frequency with which it comes into contact with the teeth. As an example, a chocolate bar eaten in one go will give one burst of potential tooth decay. However, that same bar broken into six and eaten spread out during the day will produce six potential attacks of tooth decay, which could do far more damage.

Here are some hints to help protect your child's teeth:

- try to confine sweets to a specific time of the day or the week
- snacking during the day is best done with savoury rather than sweet food
- try to discourage a sweet tooth by not adding sugar to foods and drinks – parents often taste baby foods and then, finding them bland, add some sugar; this can give the child a very strong liking for overly sweet food
- watch how much of the family budget is spent on confectionery; if it is more than £1-2 per week the child is probably eating too many sweets
- sticky or chewy sweets are probably worse than boiled sweets as they hang around the mouth longer, so can cause more damage
- never let a baby or small child go to sleep with a bottle or dummy with anything sweet in it, even dilute fruit juice, as a night-time comforter – this can cause a particularly severe form of decay called bottle decay.

Strengthening the teeth

The only proven way of making tooth enamel more resistant is by the use of fluoride, which makes teeth far less prone to cavities. It also promotes healing (remineralisation) of early cavities. It gets into the tooth enamel in several ways.

The most effective method is to drink water which has fluoride present in it, either naturally or added by the water authority. Children living in all these areas have a much lower incidence of tooth decay. (Some areas have no fluoride in the water.) This way, the fluoride is taken into the tooth enamel while the teeth are still being formed beneath the gums.

A slightly less effective method is for fluoride to be put on to the enamel after it has formed. Fluoride is added to most brands of toothpaste and the huge decrease in dental decay in the last thirty years is thought to be due largely to the introduction and use of fluoride toothpastes. Fluoride can also be put on to the teeth by the dentist as a concentrated gel or varnish. At home you can use a fluoride rinse, or fluoride tablets or drops (but see 'Some words of caution'). These work in two ways: the fluoride swallowed will strengthen any developing teeth and the tablet slowly dissolving will strengthen teeth that are already in the mouth.

SOME WORDS OF CAUTION

- Too much fluoride can cause fluorosis, which can produce effects ranging from minor enamel defects to severe discolouring (mottling) of the teeth.
- You need to be aware of the total amount of fluoride being taken from all sources. Your water authority will let you know the levels of fluoride in your drinking water.
- Use only a pea-sized amount of children's low-dose fluoride toothpaste but don't rinse out. The small amount of swallowed toothpaste will help developing teeth and not rinsing will keep the fluoride in contact with the teeth for longer where it can be more beneficial. Always follow the manufacturer's guidelines and if in doubt, consult your dentist.

Visits to the dentist

Register your child with a dentist very early on, even before his or her milk teeth are through. Make sure you are with a dentist who enjoys seeing children (most do). The best way to find a dentist is through personal recommendation. Alternatively, try the phone book or the dental list from your local health authority. Ask the dentist or the staff about the kind of services the practice provides, especially about preventative care. If you are nervous of dentists, make your child a separate appointment – you do not want them to learn fear from you. Changing dentists is straightforward, as far as children – who are fee-exempt – are concerned: simply take them to another one (their parents may have greater difficulty transferring if they want to continue as NHS patients). Unlike doctors, dentists can see patients irrespective of where they live.

Treatment

Most dentists now wear latex gloves as a precaution against the transfer of blood-borne diseases.

Most dentistry to children's teeth in the UK takes the form of fillings, although if a tooth is too badly damaged it may need to be taken out. 'Silver fillings' are usually made of mercury amalgam. Although mercury is a potentially toxic material and some mercury from fillings does enter the body, the amounts involved are very small compared to mercury found in natural sources. There is little evidence that it does any harm except in rare cases of mercury allergy. It is not known if any of the non-mercury alternatives are any safer. Most authorities consider mercury to be harmless, but if you are worried speak to your dentist.

If the dentist feels that an injection is necessary – not all fillings require one – remember that modern anaesthetics are virtually painless and your child may hardly realise that he or she has had one. Be careful not to let your child chew his or her lip while it is numb.

X-rays

Dental x-rays are one of the most useful ways for dentists to examine the areas which cannot be seen by just looking, such as small cavities which would otherwise not be found until they were much larger. Other x-ray pictures can show whether the teeth are developing correctly and that the jaws are growing properly. Modern dental x-rays use very low doses of radiation (approximately the same amount that a child would receive by flying abroad on holiday), so it is not usually necessary to protect a child with a lead apron. However, all radiation is potentially dangerous, so if you do not wish your child to be x-rayed, let your dentist know, bearing in mind that he or she may fail to detect a problem until it has grown much larger.

NHS or private dental treatment

The vast majority of children are treated under the NHS. Even those dentists who treat adults only privately will treat children under the NHS, where children's treatment is free. Under the NHS, the dentist must provide only the least expensive treatment option. However, some dentists feel that these financial constraints do not allow them to spend sufficient time with the children under their care, or they may want to use techniques or materials that are different from the ones they are obliged to use under the NHS. For these reasons your dentist may recommend private treatment or a combination of the two.

Private treatment may be paid for either by fees paid directly to the dentist or by a monthly payments scheme provided by a dental insurance plan. Find out about the method of payment before your child undertakes any treatment.

The dental team

Other professionals on the dental team may include the dental hygienist and the dental health educator. Some practices may charge a private fee for the preventative services offered by these members of the team. Make sure that you know beforehand what (if any) charges will be involved.

The community dental service

This service, normally run out of local clinics, is another provider of dental care. The clinics operate entirely within the NHS and may be contacted through your local health authority. This is also the part of the NHS that ensures that every child receives a dental examination at school.

Complaints

If you have any complaint about your child's care, the first person to approach is the dentist. All NHS practices have an in-house complaints procedure which should be able to resolve most problems amicably. If you are unhappy with the dentist's response, the next step is to take up the matter with your local health authority. The community health council may assist you with a complaint about treatment under the NHS. Further redress can be brought by bringing a civil case in a court of law or through the professional body which regulates the dental profession, the General Dental Council.*

In the case of private treatment, if you are unable to get satisfaction through the dentist himself or herself, the only redress available is through the courts.

Dental problems

See Chapter 4 for how to help a teething baby. Some other common problems affecting teeth and gums are dealt with below.

Orthodontics

Most children, especially as they begin to lose their milk teeth and get their permanent teeth, develop crooked teeth. One reason for this is simply that the adult teeth erupt at their full size but the mouth is not yet big enough for them, so they come through crowded as the only way of fitting in. There may also be problems of congenitally missing teeth, teeth that fail to erupt or teeth that erupt in the wrong place.

The jaws can also fail to develop adequately. Regular examinations are the best way of monitoring the development of the teeth and jaws. Crooked teeth will often correct themselves with time, but sometimes treatment is required. The treatment may involve extracting teeth to create more space and fitting a brace on to the ones that are left. This treatment may be carried out by the child's dentist, by an orthodontist, or by both working in consultation.

Braces may be either removable (a plastic plate worn in the mouth) or fixed (wires bonded to the teeth). Sometimes a special brace may be required to alter the rate of growth of the jaws so that the face develops properly (dento-facial orthopaedics). Very severe cases may even require surgery. Many children are keen to wear braces to be like their friends; and many braces come in different colours, so children can, for instance, choose the colour of their favourite football team.

Injuries

The first dental injury commonly occurs when a toddler falls and damages a front tooth. This often results in nothing more serious than the tooth darkening, but it is best to have any injury of this nature checked by your dentist. Very occasionally, the developing permanent tooth in the gum may be damaged as a result of injury. If a permanent tooth is broken, the child needs to see the dentist as soon as possible.

A small injury may need no more than reassurance and monitoring, but a more severe breakage may require some kind of repair treatment. If a permanent tooth is totally knocked out it should be gently cleaned if it is dirty and pushed back into the socket as soon as possible. If an adult is unable to do this, the child should be taken to the dentist immediately with the tooth kept moist either inside the child's cheek or in some milk. The sooner the tooth is fixed back in, the better are the chances of success (but they are not great).

Contact sports are a common cause of dental injuries, so a custom-made gum shield should be worn. They are available in a wide range of bright colours.

Acid erosion

A relatively new problem that is arising over children's teeth is for them to be dissolved away by food containing acid. Many popular – and healthy – foods contain a high level of acid. Oranges contain citric acid, apples contain malic acid, diet cola phosphoric acid, yoghurt lactic acid – even fizzy water contains carbonic acid. The extent of this problem and its future impact cannot be gauged but dentists are beginning to see youngsters who have no cavities in their teeth, yet who are losing the irreplaceable enamel from their teeth.

The current advice is not to brush your teeth within an hour of eating anything with a high acid content. This allows the saliva in the mouth to re-harden any enamel that may have been softened by the acid.

Mouth ulcers

Ulcers are shallow craters which can occasionally appear on the inner linings of the mouth or on the tongue. The cause is often unknown. These aphthous ulcers tend to be sore and distressing, and children may not want to eat or to brush their teeth. Aphthous ulcers can recur with no predictable pattern.

Sometimes a virus can cause mouth ulcers – the herpes virus is often implicated. Both types of ulcer tend to heal in a few days.

Simple antiseptic mouth washes, the application of soothing gels and pain relief such as paracetamol may be needed. Though children may go off their food, it's important for them to drink fluids. You could try giving them soft or liquidised food which might be easier to swallow. If the child is not drinking enough fluids or is just plain miserable, or if the ulcers persist, it would be sensible to see the doctor.

Thrush in the mouth

This is commonly seen in young babies and represents an overgrowth in the mouth of the yeast organism (the same one that causes vaginal thrush). The mouth is coated with white spots and may be sore. If treatment is needed anti-fungal drops often be prescribed. Most parents of young babies initially seek advice from their GP.

Gum disease

Many forms of gum disease which can become a serious problem in adult life start as a minor problem in childhood. The most common is gingivitis, in which the gums become red, inflamed and bleed easily. It is usually caused by a failure to clean the plaque from the teeth well enough or often enough. It is best prevented by maintaining high standards of oral hygiene. If hard scale (calculus) is also building up on the teeth and irritating the gums, this will need to be professionally removed by the dentist or hygienist.

Toothache

The most common cause of toothache is dental decay in a tooth. If the cavity is particularly deep, the tooth can develop a dental abscess. Treatment should be sought from the dentist at the first sign of any problem. Some cavities can be treated with fillings but larger ones may require the tooth to be extracted. Once again, it is much better to try to prevent the problem from developing in the first place.

CHAPTER 8

GETTING THE BEST MEDICAL CARE FOR YOUR CHILD

LIKE every other health service in the world, the National Health Service is called upon to deliver more than its resources can provide. Some services – assisted conception, for example – are no longer available under the NHS in certain areas, but this is the exception rather than the rule, and for children under 12 the NHS offers a pretty comprehensive service at a reasonably high standard. But the NHS is a vast organisation and standards can vary from one region to another, so to get the best from it for you and your family it is important to know a little about how the system works.

Family doctors (GPs)

As a parent you are probably registered with a doctor already. If you have a new baby, it is likely that you will want the child to be registered with the same GP as yourself. This is not essential, but it can help the doctor to treat young patients if he or she is familiar with the family medical history and circumstances. If the parents are registered with different practices, as is often the case for historical reasons, the time when you are registering your new baby may be a good opportunity to consider moving the whole family to the same practice.

Finding a doctor

Most practices cover a well-defined geographical area and will not take patients who live beyond its boundaries. You will have a greater choice of doctors if you live in an urban area; in some rural areas you will have little or none.

If you are new to an area, it is worth asking neighbours which practice they attend and how happy are they with the service they receive. Another useful source of information may be the local pharmacy, whose staff are likely to have regular dealings with the local doctors.

You could also ask the local health authority/board, which administers family doctor services, for information about GP services in your area. The phone number can be found in the local phone book.

Doctors can refuse to let a prospective patient register with them and can remove anyone from their list without having to give a reason. A doctor is obliged to accept a patient only if he or she has had difficulty in finding a doctor and has therefore been allocated to one by the health authority/board. Everyone has the right to be registered with a GP and health authorities/boards have a duty to find you a doctor if you have had problems in doing so yourself.

No doctor should refuse to administer emergency or other urgent treatment when no one else is available to treat a patient.

Once you have found a local GP who is willing to take you and your family on to his or her list, all you have to do is register by completing some straightforward forms.

Changing your doctor

If you have a disagreement with your current doctor or you are just unhappy with the current level of service, you can change doctors. You do not need to give a reason; nor do you require the permission of the previous doctor. Just turn up at the new practice, with your NHS card if you have it, and ask if you can be taken on. You fill in the registration form and then the practice will arrange your new-patient health check, so that they can get to know you.

Your health authority/board will transfer your medical records from your old GP to the new one and send you a new medical card.

What aspects of a GP's practice are important to you?

GP practices do not all offer the same services to patients, so it is worth finding out what yours offers for babies and children and, if there are special baby clinics, when they are held. Basic information will be contained in the practice leaflet (ask the receptionist for the latest version), though it may be limited to clinic times and a brief description of the practice. Many family doctors offer a full range of services including immunisations and child health surveillance (see Chapters 3 and 4).

Any of the following aspects of a GP's practice may be important to you:

- Attitude of the practice team to sick babies and children. Ask other mothers who are registered with the practice (or pregnant women attending the ante-natal clinic who have other children looked after by the practice members) how quickly their children are seen when they are ill and whether the doctors, in particular, seem confident and knowledgeable where babies and children are concerned.
- The health visitor and practice nurse: for routine child care you will probably have minimal contact with the GP. The health visitor will be your key contact, while the practice nurse may be the one who administers vaccinations. Rapport with these members of the team, and confidence in what they do, is important.
- Attitude of the rest of the team, including the receptionists, who are commonly the first point of contact when you need to see a doctor.
- The GP's style: many patients want information about their own health problems and those of their children and wish to be involved in decisions. Others are happy for the doctor to decide what is best and then be told of this.
- The age and sex of the GP.
- The attitude of the doctor to complementary therapies.
- Any special interest or expertise that the GP may have, such as wide experience in treating asthma, eczema or diabetes, for instance, which may be of relevance to your family.
- The practice itself, and the way it is run. Its location will be a prime consideration, particularly if you have young children and no car. The quality of the premises: is there any privacy in the reception area? Are there toys in the waiting room? There should be enough space to accommodate a full surgery session and ideally an isolation area where a child with a suspected infectious disease can wait during a busy surgery.

- Number of doctors working in the practice: many GPs work in group practices. Two of the advantages of this are that it gives patients a choice of doctors to see, and that a second opinion can be obtained within the practice.
- Whether the practice runs an appointment-only system, or has walk-in surgeries.
- How the practice copes with out-of-hours care. NHS family doctors have a contractual obligation to provide care round the clock. Many now have extended rotas using cover from other practices, although in certain rural areas doctors who practise on their own still cope with all the out-of-hours care themselves, except when illness or holidays make this impossible. Some family doctors offer an out-of-hours service which includes an emergency centre that people can attend rather than waiting for a doctor to call. Others use a commercial deputising service, or work with other practices on a co-operative basis. The out-of-hours number should be on the practice leaflet, but if you are unsure which one to use check with the practice manager or receptionist.

If ever you are unhappy about the level of service you are getting from your doctor, say something. Most doctors are much more responsive to the needs of their patients than they used to be.

Getting the best from your GP

Young families, especially those with young children, tend to be frequent users of their GP's practice.

Parents, especially if they are under stress, often seek home visits for their children, but in many cases there is no reason why the child cannot be taken to the doctor's surgery, especially if transport is available or can be arranged.

Visiting the surgery

Some parents worry about taking their child to the doctor unnecessarily. Young children may not be able to describe what is wrong with them, their temperatures may fluctuate within a short space of time, and they may be ill one moment and perfectly well an hour later. Pain can also be short-lived. But if you are seriously concerned, that is reason enough for taking your child to the doctor; the vast majority of doctors and their staff will understand, even if the problem turns out to be insignificant. After all, many of them are parents themselves and know what it is like to be anxious about a sick child.

If you have to take an ailing child to the surgery:

- telephone first, and warn the receptionist if you think the child is infectious
- once you are there, ask the receptionist to try to minimise the delay between arrival and seeing the doctor
- if the child is likely to be infectious ask if you can sit in an area away from the other patients or to be seen at the beginning or end of the surgery
- if you feel you are waiting an unreasonable length of time to see the doctor, speak to the receptionist
- always try to keep an appointment; if you cannot, let the surgery know, so that another patient can take up the slot.

The hospital service

While GPs offer 'primary care', being the first port of call for patients, the service provided by hospitals is sometimes described as secondary care.

Some cities have specialised children's hospitals, or children's units that represent a sizeable department of a general hospital. A child's first contact with the hospital service could be as a casualty. Children are heavy users of accident and emergency (formerly casualty) departments, simply because they are more prone to injuries; many are referred to these units by their GP.

Some accident and emergency units are more child-friendly than others. Ideally, an accident and emergency department should have a separate children's area, with a few toys, but the users of such facilities are hardly likely to be in a position to pick and choose which they attend.

Occasionally, acute medical or surgical children's problems are seen in the accident and emergency department, where they are either handled by the accident and emergency staff or referred to other specialist teams within the hospital.

Sometimes the GP will make an outpatient appointment for a child to be seen by a doctor specialising in childhood diseases (a paediatrician), a paediatric surgeon or other specialist: this is known as a referral.

A GP may refer a child to a specialist because he or she is unable to solve a problem, wants an expert second opinion for peace of mind, or, perhaps, needs to satisfy an unhappy parent that the right medical decisions are being made. If you want a referral to a specialist, discuss the matter with your doctor and try not to be too anxious that it will be seen as implied criticism of his or her handling of the situation. More often than not, the doctor will agree to your request.

Visiting the outpatient clinic

Before you take your child to the outpatient clinic, discuss with your GP the reasons for the referral and what the GP hopes the consultation with the specialist will produce. Write down any questions you want to ask – otherwise, you may find that anxiety causes you to forget them – and ask about any unfamiliar words or phrases until you are sure you understand what they mean.

Do not be disappointed if, as often happens, a member of the consultant's team rather than the consultant in person sees your child, but ask to speak to the specialist if you feel unhappy about this.

Children can find the experience of a hospital visit unsettling, even if both parents are there, so explain beforehand what is going to happen and why. Some parents try to turn it into a game to reduce the apprehension.

Be clear about what tests, if any, are going to be undertaken, the reasons behind them and what exactly is involved. Also, be sure to find out how the results will be communicated to you.

Sometimes blood tests are needed, which some children find distressing. If this applies to yours, you may be able to use a cream beforehand, available on prescription, which acts as a local anaesthetic on the skin.

At the end of the consultation clarify what is to happen next and any arrangements for further appointments, or hospital admittance.

Staying in hospital

Many surgical procedures can be carried out as day cases so that the disruption to the family's routine is minimised. Inpatient stays are kept to as short a time as possible but if it becomes necessary for your child to stay overnight or longer there is much that can be done to relieve the fear and worry that this may cause.

Try to prepare your child for the experience. Many young children will have little idea why they have to go to hospital. They may find it difficult to make the connection between previous clinic visits and actually staying in hospital away from their usual surroundings. Explain the best way you can about what is going to happen.

At the same time be truthful. If the child asks if the treatment is going to hurt, and it will (you will know either way from the questions you have asked at the outpatient appointments), then be honest and say that it may do. It may help you to read up about your child's problem beforehand, too.

Try to describe what the ward will be like and the role of the doctors and nurses, perhaps with the help of pictures or your own drawings. You may be able to speak to the staff of the ward where the child will be staying, and to arrange a pre-admission visit so that your child will not be coming to a completely unfamiliar environment when admission time approaches.

Involve him or her in the process of packing and bring a few favourite toys. The hospital may be able to offer facilities for accommodation so that you can stay there with your child, which will probably make the experience much easier for the child, especially if you are able to get involved with some aspects of his or her care.

Adolescent children should have the choice of going either to a children's or an adult ward.

If your child needs a long period of hospitalisation some form of education may be required during this time. If necessary, visiting teachers can be organised so that the child does not fall too far behind.

If things go wrong

Complaining is something that most people find difficult, but if you have a valid reason for wanting to complain about how the care of your child has been handled, follow these guidelines.

It is important to think about what you want to achieve by complaining. Many people want someone to say they are sorry, explain exactly what happened and why, and say what will be done to stop it happening to others. Your best bet in most cases is to start with the NHS complaints system: it can give you an apology and details of what the GP or health authority/board will do to ensure the reason for complaint will not happen again.

A complaint about your GP

If you are unhappy about the care or treatment you or your child has been given, or the way the practice is organised, the first step is to raise your concern with your GP, the practice manager, the receptionist or the practice nurse. Being open and honest at the time about how you feel and what you want can stop a small grumble growing into a serious grievance. The majority of problems are caused by a breakdown in communication.

The NHS system covers only GPs' contractual obligations to patients, so only complaints such as failing to visit or delays in diagnosing or giving treatment are covered. If you think your GP has behaved unethically, unprofessionally or imcompetently, complain directly to his or her professional body, the General Medical Council.* The GMC can strike a GP off the register of doctors, limit what he or she can do, or suspend him or her from practising altogether.

If you have a complaint relating to professional conduct by a nurse, midwife or health visitor, you can complain to the UK Central Council for Nursing, Midwifery and Health Visiting.*

If you want compensation for what has happened to your child, you will probably have to take legal action, which could be time-consuming and expensive (see 'Seeking compensation through the courts', below).

The NHS complaints procedure

If you want assistance over complaining, your local Community Health Council will be able to help. The Councils represent patients' interests on many levels and can represent you at meetings, for instance. To obtain the address of your local Council, contact your local health authority/board, or the Association of Community Health Councils for England and Wales,* or look in the phone book.

Stage 1: local resolution

All GPs have a staff member who co-ordinates a system that receives, sorts and responds to complaints, perhaps a GP, the practice manager or nurse – the practice leaflet should indicate who is responsible. If you prefer, telephone or write to the complaints manager at your local health authority/board. Make your complaint in writing within six months of the event, if possible, or within a year at most. Your letter should be acknowledged within two working days.

Next there will be a full investigation. You should get a letter explaining what happened within ten working days of making your complaint, an apology if appropriate, details of what action has been taken and information on how to take things further if you want to.

Stage 2: independent review panel

If you are not satisfied with the results of the local resolution, ask your health authority for an independent panel to be set up to review the complaint. You need to do this within 28 days of your reply from the practice: the complaints manager should tell you whom to contact. You will be asked to explain in writing why you are not satisfied. Your Community Health Council can give you free help and support in making a complaint.

A *convenor* from the health authority decides whether or not to set up a panel, and you should be told about this decision within ten working days. The panel will consist of the convenor and two independent lay people, usually aided by an independent medical assessor. There won't be a formal hearing, but the panel will gather evidence from you as well as the GP, and you might be interviewed.

The investigation should be over within three months, and you should get a copy of the draft report to comment on. The final report will be sent to you, to the GP and to anyone else involved. It should explain what happened, include an apology if relevant and make recommendations to the GP or the practice. The panel does not have the power to discipline a GP or give any compensation.

The ombudsman (Health Service Commissioner)

If a panel is not set up or if you are still not satisfied, you can appeal in writing to the ombudsman (Health Service

Commissioner).★ He or she might ask the practice to investigate the complaint again. Write to the ombudsman saying why you are unhappy with the way things have gone. You do not have the absolute right to an ombudsman's investigation. If an investigation does go ahead, it will be very thorough and will make recommendations to prevent the same problem happening again.

The ombudsman will not usually investigate if you are seeking financial compensation through the courts; indeed, any part of the investigative process will stop if you are taking legal action.

A complaint about hospital treatment

If your complaint relates to hospital treatment that your child has received, you should if possible start by telling someone close to the cause of your complaint (a doctor, nurse or receptionist, for example). If you prefer to speak to someone who has not been involved in your child's treatment, telephone or write to the NHS trust hospital's complaints manager, or general manager of the hospital or clinic, or the chief executive in the case of an NHS trust, and send a copy to the general manager of the health authority/board.

As well as your child's name, supply his or her date of birth or hospital number, quote the date of the incident, the names of the staff involved (or describe them if you do not know their names) and the main points of the case, stating clearly what you want investigated. Also state what you want to happen as a result – action by staff to sort out your problem, an apology, improved services for others, or perhaps an explanation (or more information) about what happened. If they would be relevant, ask to see your child's medical records.

Your complaint will be investigated, and the Patient's Charter guarantees you a prompt response from the trust's chief executive.

Most complaints are dealt with under this procedure, but if you are still not satisfied you can request a further review, which may mean that an independent review panel is set up – this is likely to include an independent clinical assessor. The panel will recommend what action should be taken to address your complaint.

For more information about the complaints procedure, as well as about operation waiting times and the Patient's Charter, call (0800) 665544. The National Health Service Confederation★ may also be able to help.

Seeking compensation through the courts

If you think your child should be financially compensated for medical negligence, you do not have to have been through the clinical complaints procedure first, but obtaining compensation will almost certainly mean taking legal action, which (for adults) must start within three years of the incident that gave rise to the complaint. In the case of children, the three-year period does not begin until they are 18, so they have until they are 21 to bring proceedings. You can obtain guidance on pursuing the claim from your local community health council or Action for Victims of Medical Accidents (AVMA);* the latter, as well as giving you free basic legal and medical advice, can refer you to a solicitor with the appropriate experience.

Claims for medical accident or negligence are not to be undertaken lightly, even if you qualify for legal aid. As well as being expensive, and likely to take a long time, such cases are difficult to prove as well as being extremely stressful. Negligence is much more than a professional misjudgement. You will need a lawyer who is experienced in medical negligence cases, and having proved the existence of negligence your lawyer will have to show that this negligence caused harm to your child.

Your solicitor will take a statement from you about what happened and discuss costs. If the matter seems worth pursuing, and you have the money to proceed or are eligible for legal aid, the solicitor will obtain the child's medical records, identify the issues and then send them to a medical expert prior to preparing a report. This will be sent with your statement and records to a barrister for advice as to the strength of the claim and on how to proceed.

If your child's case is sufficiently strong, the health authority (or other defendant) may settle your claim out of court.

Other avenues for complaint

Taking your complaint through the NHS procedure does not prohibit you from complaining to your local councillor or MP. For example, a complaint about maladministration could be taken to your local government ombudsman. Forms for this purpose are available from council offices and Citizens Advice Bureaux, as well as from the local government ombudsman.

Private medical care

We all want the best for our family and especially for our children, so when we hear of the woes of the National Health Service, naturally we want to be able to consider the private sector. For most people that means taking out some form of insurance policy to cover the possibility of needing private care. You don't necessarily need to have private health insurance but the costs of private health care can be steep.

The initial consultation with a specialist may not be terribly expensive, perhaps £50–£100. However, further tests, inpatient stays with possible surgery and the follow-up care can run up a big bill. This may be more than many families can afford and that is where an insurance policy comes into its own. There is a huge range of policies to suit almost every need; if you are considering taking one out, discuss it with an independent financial adviser.

The **advantages** of private health care – for both children and adults – are:

- short waiting times before you are seen by the specialist
- seeing the specialist rather than one of his or her team or junior staff
- spending more time with the specialist and gaining a better understanding of the problem
- continuity of care: seeing the same person each time
- often a choice of appointment times
- inpatient stays tend to be in private rooms with good accommodation and catering facilities.

Of course, there are **disadvantages**, not least the cost of either the insurance premium or the direct cost of the private health care. In addition, insured private health care is not always comprehensive. Many policies do not cover family doctor services, complementary therapy and certain medical areas such as childbirth. Furthermore, any pre-existing conditions that you know about when you take out the policy may not be covered.

In addition, private hospitals tend to be in urban areas, and many are small, without the wide range of staff and facilities available on the same premises that most NHS hospitals can offer. Emergency treatment may not be available quite as quickly as at NHS hospitals. These caveats do not apply to all private hospitals.

You might therefore want the option of using either type of medical care for you and your family.

If you want to consider private treatment for your child, your own GP is in a excellent position to advise you of the local situation when comparing public to private health care. He or she will have no financial interest in your choice, and should be able to advise you about approximate waiting times and the appropriateness of using either service.

A complaint about private treatment

Whereas a serious NHS complaint could lead to your suing the hospital or the health authority/board, in the private sector you have to sue the practitioner personally because the doctor probably works independently, rather than being an employee of the private hospital or clinic where he or she works.

First, you have to establish that medical negligence or an accident occurred, or that a breach of contract occurred – or both. Your rights under the Supply of Goods and Services Act 1982 (common law in Scotland) are to receive a service that has been carried out with reasonable skill and care, within a 'reasonable time' where no time limit has been fixed, and for a 'reasonable charge' where no charge has been agreed in advance.

If you feel strongly that the private treatment your child received was unsatisfactory you could initially withhold payment. Thereafter, you have the option of starting court action (see above under 'Seeking compensation through the courts' for where to obtain initial advice and how to proceed if you feel your child's case is strong enough to pursue).

If you are in a private insurance scheme you could ask the insurance company, before treatment starts, whether it is prepared to send the payment cheque to you rather than to the hospital or doctor concerned.

CHAPTER 9

A-Z OF ILLNESSES AND SYMPTOMS

THIS section describes in simple terms the common and not-so-common illnesses and ailments that affect children. It is not meant to be a substitute for proper medical advice – the same, of course, applies to the rest of the book. If you cannot immediately find a condition in the A-Z, it may well be covered in another section – see the Index.

Allergy

What is it?

An allergy is a sensitivity to a substance which is harmless to most people. Conditions associated with allergies include hay fever, some types of conjunctivitis, asthma, eczema, food reactions and anaphylaxis (see page 43). As a rule, patients with allergic conditions, who are sometimes called atopic, have in common an inherited predisposition to develop hypersensitivity to inhaled and ingested substances (allergens) that are harmless to people who are not atopic.

Food allergy may contribute to symptoms of eczema in infants and young children while hay fever is generally induced by wind-borne pollen. Asthma is another condition caused by an allergic response: asthma attacks may be triggered by exposure to certain allergens, such as the house dust mite which lives in carpets, bedding and soft furnishings, to which the airways have developed increased sensitivity, causing inflammation and obstruction of the airways.

Food allergies in infancy are often related to cow's milk. This need not be milk from the milkman: artificially produced infant formula is a modified form of cow's milk that has been altered to make it approximately equivalent to breast milk in respect of fats, proteins and carbohydrate. But a baby's stomach is genetically designed to work with his or her own mother's milk and anything else is foreign. See also Chapter 5.

Eczema can also be caused by an allergic reaction on the skin – the terms eczema and dermatitis (inflammation of the skin) are often used interchangeably. Eczema is a superficial skin inflammation, characterised by little blisters, redness, swelling, oozing, crusting, scaling and usually itching. Scratching at the sore area often opens the way to infection.

What action should I take?

Treatment varies depending on the cause. For specific conditions you may want to seek medical advice. Trying to avoid the allergen would be ideal but is not always practical. It is very difficult, for example, to banish house dust mites, but sometimes reducing their numbers with regular damp dusting may help.

What should I expect?

There are a multitude of treatments for allergies: some are available from the doctor, while others can be bought without a prescription from the pharmacist. Oral antihistamines relieve most symptoms, and topical treatments such as calamine lotion may help to soothe the itch of allergic reactions. Pseudoephedrine (a decongestant) is also available in many antihistamine-decongestant preparations. If antihistamines prove unsatisfactory, sodium cromoglycate preparations may be given by nasal spray. When antihistamines inadequately relieve nasal symptoms, a steroid nose spray is usually effective. Very severe symptoms may require a short course of oral steroids. This may be justified before important exams or an event such as a family wedding.

Many children grow out of their allergies and by the time they reach adulthood have few if any allergic problems.

What else can I do?

Read the separate entries for asthma (page 151) and eczema (page 184).

WHAT TO DO IN AN EMERGENCY

Very rarely a child can experience a life-threatening allergic reaction. This is called anaphylaxis – see page 43.

Appendicitis

What is it?

Appendicitis is inflammation of the appendix, a blind-ending tube which comes out of the first part of the large intestine. Looking from the outside, the appendix is in the lower part of the abdomen, just above the right hip. In certain animals the appendix has some digestive functions, but in humans it is a redundant piece of tissue; it sometimes causes problems which may require surgery. Appendicitis can occur in adults but is particularly common between the ages of 8 and 14. It is rare in the under-two age group.

The sequence of events which leads to appendicitis is likely to start with a blockage in the appendix cavity, in which some of the bowel contents flowing through the intestines may be caught up. The inner lining of the appendix becomes inflamed; eventually this inflammation spreads through the whole thickness of the appendix. The blood vessels which supply the appendix form clots, causing the whole appendix to start to disintegrate. It is at this point that the bowel contents and bacteria can escape to the rest of the abdomen, which may lead to widespread inflammation called peritonitis. The child can become quite severely ill.

What action should I take?

Children can have numerous episodes of tummy pain and it is very difficult to identify appendicitis, particularly in the early stages. Even experienced doctors can easily get this diagnosis wrong. When your child starts complaining about tummy ache, try giving him or her a hot-water bottle to cuddle. If he or she is in obvious distress or the pain has persisted for several hours, think about getting medical advice. If your child is obviously unwell with tummy pain, take him or her to the nearest accident and emergency department.

What should I expect?

The main symptom is usually pain in the lower right-hand side of the abdomen. Often children with appendicitis have a temperature, feel nauseous and may actually be sick, and prefer to lie still. The right-hand part of the lower tummy will feel tender; the doctor will try to confirm this when he or she examines the child. If the appendix has ruptured and peritonitis has set in, the whole abdomen will be painful.

After the doctor has made a tentative diagnosis of appendicitis, the child is normally referred to hospital so that the diagnosis can be confirmed and the child can be prepared for an operation. Unfortunately, there is no specific test for appendicitis. However, tests may be performed to rule out other conditions which can simulate appendicitis, such as urine infections. If there is reasonable evidence to suggest appendicitis, a simple operation will be performed to remove the appendix. Even if the appendix is found to be normal during surgery, it will probably be removed anyway to avoid future problems. People can safely live without their appendix and suffer no long-term effects when it is removed.

What else can I do?

When your child is in pain but a diagnosis has not yet been made, it can be confusing and worrying for all of you. Even so, it is important to be positive and reassuring to your child. If appendicitis is a possibility, check with the medical or nursing staff whether your child may have a drink or something to eat. Make sure that he or she is given enough pain relief before and after the operation.

After the operation the child should get up and about as soon as possible, and where no complications arise he or she should be home in about two to three days. Children usually bounce back pretty quickly and you can start giving them their normal diet as soon as they ask for it. They should be back to school in a couple of weeks.

Arthritis

What is it?

Arthritis means inflammation of the joints. Many people tend to accept arthritis as a natural consequence of ageing but are astonished to hear that children can suffer from arthritis too. The actual cause remains unclear, although genetic (inherited) factors are likely to be involved.

It was a Dr Still who first recognised the condition we now know as juvenile chronic arthritis, in the late nineteenth century. The condition is sometimes called Still's disease or juvenile rheumatoid arthritis but these names are rather outdated now. Although it is not common, juvenile chronic arthritis can cause a child a great deal of disability.

What action should I take?

It depends on the type of arthritis, but any child with a swollen joint should be assessed by a doctor. Apart from confirming the diagnosis, the doctor will want to make sure there is no infection in the joint. This can be done by taking a sample of the fluid from around the swollen joint and sending it off to the laboratory for analysis.

When juvenile chronic arthritis is diagnosed, the parents should be closely involved in all the various aspects of the child's care. In particular, it is important to liaise with the educational authorities as schooling may be adversely affected, particularly when the child may need periods of absence. Although swimming is a suitable activity, certain sports may not be appropriate for children with arthritis. Despite these limitations, try not to overprotect children with chronic arthritis. Find out what they are capable of and help them to achieve their potential.

Supplement whatever information you glean from health professionals by joining a self-help group such as Young Arthritis Care.★

What should I expect?

There are different types of juvenile arthritis and many of their symptoms overlap. A few large joints, such as the knee, or smaller joints, such as the feet and hands, may be affected. The joint may be hot, swollen, red and stiff. If the lower limbs are involved the child may limp. Sometimes the child can be generally unwell with a temperature, swollen glands and a rash, so at the outset arthritis can easily be confused with an infectious illness.

Arthritis in children is a chronic condition punctuated with numerous episodes of acute flare-ups. During the painful episodes your child may need a splint on a badly affected joint to give relief from pain and to stop the joints becoming deformed. Physiotherapists and occupational therapists may have a role to play in helping your child to recover after a bad attack. Drug treatment can also help: anti-inflammatory drugs and steroids may help relieve the symptoms but they can have side effects. Steroids in particular can cause thinning of the bones – osteoporosis – and may impair growth when they are taken over a long period. Steroid injections in the joints provide short-term pain relief without the side effects of steroid tablets.

The outlook for a child diagnosed with juvenile chronic arthritis is generally quite good. Most children get better and are left with very little, if any, disability. Only a small proportion go on to develop adult types of arthritis.

What else can I do?
Acupuncture, herbal medicine and homeopathy can be useful, but always keep your GP informed. It may well be that your GP or paediatrician can recommend an appropriate practitioner.

You may be entitled to certain welfare benefits to help with the care that your child requires – check with the social services, the hospital social worker or the local Citizens Advice Bureau.

Asthma

What is it?
Asthma is a very common condition of the airways and lungs which affects about one in seven children in the UK. The disease is thought to have become more common in recent years. This may be a real increase or it may just be that doctors are getting better at recognising and diagnosing it. Asthma is particularly difficult to diagnose in children – symptoms such as coughing and wheezing are hallmarks of a number of respiratory conditions. Asthma occurs when the airways which allow air to flow to and from the lungs narrow. The degree of narrowing can vary rapidly over a relatively short period of time but it can be reversed by treatment or as the problem settles on its own. However, treatment does not actually cure the condition, it just suppresses it, and even if the

condition ultimately improves by itself, there is a reasonable risk of relapse.

The narrowing is caused by an inflammation of the airways in the lung, increased mucus production, and contraction of the muscles surrounding the tube walls. In some cases a link is thought to exist with allergic conditions. Asthma is commonly found in children with other disorders which have an allergic basis, such as hay fever and eczema. It has an entirely physical basis and is not caused by 'nerves', although an emotional crisis can set off an asthma attack.

In most cases, asthma is a condition which comes and goes – children should be well between attacks. The symptoms of asthma – wheezing, breathlessness and coughing – can be triggered by viral or bacterial infection; exercise, particularly when breathing in cold air; or by allergies to the house dust mite or pets. Asthma symptoms often flare up during the early hours of the morning and the persistent cough – with or without wheezing – often interrupts sleep. Severe asthma attacks can be frightening for both parents and children. If your child has a major problem with breathing, your doctor may suggest that he or she is admitted to hospital. Without treatment, asthma can be fatal.

What action should I take?

When a child has a persistent cough or problem with wheezing, parents should be aware that asthma is a possibility and make an appointment to see the doctor. No specific test has been devised that will confirm or exclude the diagnosis of asthma and many doctors will use a therapeutic trial to see whether the symptoms respond. The signs that suggest asthma include:

- persistent cough
- a family history of asthma or allergic conditions (such as hay fever or eczema)
- coughing that is worse at night
- coughing and wheezing that get worse after running about
- getting out of breath easily and finding it difficult to keep up with friends during physical activity.

What should I expect?

Before examining your child, the GP will ask you questions about what signs you have noticed. He or she may find when listening to the child's chest that it is clear, even if the child is suffering from asthma. The doctor may carry out a 'peak flow' test: the child is told to take a deep breath and then blow hard into a hollow tube to blast a little button down towards the end of the cylinder. The distance the button travels can be read off against a scale and translated into a number which indicates the volume of air blown out. This information can easily be measured regularly and a trend established. The doctor may give you a prescription for a peak flow meter so that you can test your child at home.

Using a peak flow meter is an integral part of measuring airway obstruction and should be performed regularly, whether or not the asthma is bad at the time: an unusually low reading could give an early warning that the airways are narrowing. It is the equivalent of using a blood pressure measuring device to check blood pressure. Once diagnosed, asthma should be regularly monitored either by the family doctor or at a hospital clinic.

Many of the treatments revolve around the use of inhalers, by which drugs are drawn into the lungs via the airways. Two types of drugs are used in inhalers:

- 'relievers', which open the airways and restore them to their normal size within minutes
- 'preventers', which are usually inhaled steroids – these drugs do not give immediate relief from symptoms but control the underlying inflammation.

The two types of medication should be used together.

The amount and type of medication should be tailored to the individual child's needs so that the asthma is well controlled. It is preferable to use inhalers rather than tablets because inhalers will deliver drugs to the site where they are needed with minimal side effects. But there is a knack to using inhalers, and not all children, particularly young children, will be able to manage them. There are several types of inhaler and adaptations so your child may need to try out the various types with different attachments before finding one that suits him or her. Usage will still need to be reviewed regularly by a doctor, nurse or health visitor. Steroid tablets or liquids are occasionally used, especially in a time of crisis. This is usually alongside, not instead of, inhalers.

Parents are often concerned when they hear the word 'steroids'. It is true that steroids are potent drugs, but in the inhaled form they are pretty safe, have a potent anti-inflammatory effect on the airways, and are unlikely to have any long-term side effects. Even so, their use needs to be monitored and reviewed regularly. Steroid tablets may be prescribed as a short, sharp course to end a bad episode of asthma, but again there should be no problem. It is only when steroid tablets are used for several weeks and months that side effects start to appear.

What else can I do?

Both children with asthma and their carers need to be involved in monitoring the disorder. Parents should check their child's peak flow regularly once he or she is above the age of six or seven. This gives an objective indication of how well the asthma is being controlled and is better than just relying on symptoms or how frequently the inhaler is used, although the latter two may also be useful indicators. It is worth charting these readings on the graph paper which comes with the peak flow meter. If your doctor has not prescribed a meter, ask for one, and use it regularly. If your child's breathing worsens at any time, take a reading. If it is lower than expected and the symptoms seem severe, this is a sign that your child needs to see the doctor. You can discuss with your doctor the thresholds below which you need to get help.

It is essential that you always have a good stock of inhalers at home, so that you never run out. Your child could also keep a spare one at school. In many cases, children's asthma is brought on by exercise, such as games at school. This kind of reaction may be pre-empted by taking a dose of the reliever type of inhaler perhaps 30 minutes or so before the exercise.

You can make sure that your child's asthma is controlled as much as possible with the conventional medical treatments, but there is usually no harm in trying complementary therapies as well. Herbal medicines may help to loosen the thickened sputum associated with asthma, and inhalations of eucalyptus are thought to be helpful. Homeopathy may have something to offer asthma sufferers – a wide range of potential therapies is available. Relaxation therapies and yoga may offer benefits too. As always, consult a qualified practitioner and never stop your child's conventional therapy without first discussing it with your GP.

WHAT TO DO IN AN EMERGENCY

Asthma can be frightening for both the child and the parents, and it is typically worse at night. If you think it is getting worse, check your child's peak flows to see if they are a lot lower than normal. Then, if your child is distressed and if the usual medication is having no effect, ring your doctor and tell him or her about the symptoms. Be prepared to take your child to the surgery quickly if necessary. If transport is a problem or the child is too ill to move, your doctor may come to your home. In either case, find out how long it will to take for you to see the doctor. If there is going to be a significant delay or the child is quite unwell, you may need to dial 999 for an ambulance or take your child to the nearest accident and emergency department.

Asthma is a potentially fatal condition which must be taken seriously. Don't be frightened to make a fuss if you feel it is necessary.

Breathing difficulties

See **asthma**, page 151; **bronchiolitis**, page 28; **congenital heart disease,** page 162; **croup**, page 168; **diphtheria**, page 178; **epiglottitis**, page 186.

Brittle nails

See **ringworm**, page 233.

Bronchitis

See **respiratory tract infection**, page 229.

Cancer

What is it?

Cancer is a new growth of tissue caused by the excessive and uncontrolled growth of abnormal cells that have the ability to invade and destroy other tissues. Cancer, which may arise from any type of cell and in any body tissue, is not a single disease but a large number of diseases classified according to the tissues involved and the type of cell where the disease originates.

Although numerous different types of cancer can arise in childhood, childhood cancer is actually very rare. Some cancers are more common than others in children.

Brain tumours

After leukaemia (see page 211) the next most common cancers in children are those that occur within the brain, particularly astrocytomas and medulloblastoma. The problem with brain tumours is that whether they are benign or malignant (which means they may spread to other places), they can do a lot of local damage just by growing in a confined space. As the skull is rigid, tumours can grow only at the expense of other structures, some of which may be vital. These cancers make their presence known usually by the pressure they put on adjacent tissues (which is why they are often referred to as space-occupying lesions). The usual symptoms include headache, visual disturbances, nausea, vomiting and changes in behaviour such as mood swings.

Doctors make the diagnosis by examining the nervous system, and by checking for swelling in the optic nerve by looking through the pupils at the back of the eyes. More specific information can be obtained from specialised scans of the brain such as computerised tomography – a computer-enhanced x-ray technique (CT scan), and magnetic resonance imaging (MRI). Both can give excellent images of what is going on inside the brain are quite safe.

Brain tumours may need an operation, with or without radiotherapy and chemotherapy. The difficulty is that the tumours are often diagnosed late and are often in parts of the brain where it is not easy to operate. The good news is that more tumours are being diagnosed earlier, and that treatment techniques are constantly being improved.

Retinoblastoma

Retinoblastoma is a malignant tumour that arises from the retina, the photosensitive lining at the back of the eye. It is very rare, occurring in only one or two out of every 30,000 babies, but it represents about 2 per cent of childhood malignancies. There may be a genetic predisposition to the disorder since about 10 per cent of children with it have a family history of retinoblastoma. The diagnosis is usually made before the child is two. If the tumour is on only one side, the eye is removed along with as much of the optic nerve as possible. This treatment is successful in 90 per cent of children when the tumour is limited to the eye. Intensive drug treatment may also be helpful, particularly if the disease has spread beyond the eyeball. When someone has retinoblastoma it is essential to test other close family members for signs of the condition.

Wilm's tumour
Also known as a nephroblastoma, this is a kidney tumour which can arise at an early age. Some genetic factors may be involved. Wilm's tumour is usually diagnosed in children under five years of age, but can occasionally be detected in older children and very rarely in adults. The diagnosis is usually prompted by finding a swelling in the abdomen. Other symptoms include abdominal pain, blood in the urine, fever, loss of appetite, nausea and vomiting. A simple ultrasound scan similar to that used in pregnancy can help make the diagnosis. A CT scan of the abdomen is helpful in determining the extent of the tumour, but as far as children are concerned it is usually carried out under general anaesthetic as it involves keeping perfectly still for long periods. The treatment involves surgical removal of the tumour followed by chemotherapy. The outlook depends on what doctors find when they look at the tumour under the microscope, how advanced it was at the time of diagnosis, and the age of the patient – the younger the better.

Neuroblastoma
This tumour is often found in the adrenal gland, which lies above the kidney and produces the hormone adrenaline. Some evidence shows that this form of cancer runs in the family. The symptoms vary depending on where the cancer starts and how far the disease has progressed, but often there is a mass in the abdomen or symptoms that the cancer has spread to the liver, the lung or the bone, especially the region of the skull around the eye. If bones are involved, the child may have bone pain. If the bone marrow is involved the child may be anaemic and may have rashes. Neuroblastoma is diagnosed using scans and laboratory tests on

blood. It is best treated by surgical removal of the tumour, often followed by chemotherapy. The outlook depends on the child's age when the condition is diagnosed – the younger the child at the time of diagnosis, the better the prospect of a cure.

Malignant melanoma
A malignant melanoma is a tumour which occurs in a pigmented area, usually the skin, but also at the back of the eyes. Malignant melanomas vary in size, shape and colour, although they are usually dark. This form of cancer can spread very rapidly and sometimes it may be fatal within months of being found. However, if malignant melanomas are spotted early enough the survival rate is extremely high. This early diagnosis and cure depend upon the child seeing a doctor as soon as the parents suspect something.

Because the incidence of melanoma is increasing, vigorous campaigns to alert the public are under way in several areas of the world. Prevention means not just avoiding sunburn but too much exposure to the sun in general, and regularly watching for any changes in the skin. The following danger signs suggest malignant changes in coloured moles:

- a change in size
- a change in colour – especially the spread of coloured pigments to surrounding normal skin
- a change in surface characteristics, consistency or shape
- signs of inflammation in the surrounding skin.

Malignant melanomas are very rare in children but can arise from large pigmented moles that are present at birth. Melanomas have to be cut out, although newer forms of therapy including chemotherapy are being developed.

Osteosarcoma – bone tumour
Osteosarcoma is the most common tumour to start in the bone and it is highly malignant, with a tendency to spread to the lungs. It is most common in people aged 10 to 20, although it can occur at any age. About half of these cancers are located around the knee but they can be found in any bone. Pain and swelling are the usual symptoms. X-ray findings vary greatly so an accurate diagnosis rests on an examination of a biopsy specimen. Treatment involves an operation with radiotherapy and/or chemotherapy either before

or afterwards. In the past a limb would have been amputated to remove the tumour, but nowadays the tumour can be cut away and the limb reconstructed. This kind of treatment has a 75 per cent success rate. Numerous clinical studies are under way to improve survival even further.

Another type of bone cancer – Ewing's sarcoma – can occur in quite young children, although the peak incidence is among people aged 10 to 20. Boys are more likely to develop it than girls. Most of the tumours develop at the ends of the long bones in the arms and legs, but any bone may be involved. Pain and swelling are the most common symptoms. Ewing's tumour tends to be extensive, sometimes affecting the entire shaft of a long bone. The diagnosis depends on a biopsy, since many other malignant bone tumours produce an identical appearance. Treatment includes various combinations of surgery, chemotherapy and radiotherapy. Currently, more than 60 per cent of people with a localised Ewing's sarcoma of the bone may be cured.

What action should I take?
Any unusual symptom that persists should be seen by a doctor. But don't get too worried: childhood cancers are relatively rare. Most family doctors will see only a few cases while they are in general practice.

What should I expect?
In most cases of childhood cancer the outlook is good, but you must be realistic and expect doctors to be very honest with you. It is important for a child with cancer to have hope, because the human mind can make a large difference to the outcome. Don't be afraid to ask for help for yourself and other family members: this is an illness that will affect the whole family. In most specialist cancer units there are specially trained people to support you through your ordeal. Remember that your GP is also there to help.

What else can I do?
Most of the diseases discussed here are rare and most GPs will have limited knowledge about them. Although you will get used to the routine and jargon used by the experts, the technical issues may be complex, so you may want to contact a self-help group. Information about the most appropriate group is likely to be avail-

able from the hospital team looking after your child. Not only will you find out more about the condition but you will also get support from other families in a similar position.

Chickenpox

What is it?

Chickenpox is one of the common childhood illnesses. It is an infection caused by a virus called *Varicella-zoster*, one of the herpes group of viruses. It is a highly infectious illness with an incubation period of about two weeks: in other words, it may be two weeks after your child has been exposed to the virus before symptoms appear. The virus can be passed on by another person infected by chickenpox or by a person suffering from shingles. (However, you cannot catch shingles from someone who has chickenpox or shingles: shingles involves the reactivation of the chickenpox virus which remains in the body, close to the spinal cord within nerve roots, even after recovery from the chickenpox illness.)

Chickenpox can occur at any age, but it is most common in children under the age of ten. There is usually a three- to four-day illness with a mild fever and headache before the characteristic spots begin to appear. These are small, itchy, fluid-filled blisters which can occur anywhere on the body. Fresh crops of spots appear over the next few days. The spots begin to break down, weep and then scab over. When all the spots have dried and scabbed over – about a week after they first appear – the child is no longer infectious. Sometimes, children have a mild illness with just a few spots, while others can be very ill with an extensive rash.

What action should I take?

The fever and headache can be treated with tepid sponging and paracetamol. The itching can be soothed with a preparation such as calamine lotion. If this is ineffective you could try antihistamine medicines, but check with your doctor or pharmacist first.

What should I expect?

In the majority of cases, chickenpox starts to clear up after about a week without too much trouble. However, there are a few complications for which you need to be on the lookout.

- Some of the spots may become red and angry-looking, weeping yellow fluid. This is a sign of a secondary bacterial infection which may need to be treated with antibiotics.
- The spots may affect sensitive areas such as the face, particularly the eyes and mouth, or the nappy area.
- On very rare occasions, chickenpox can lead to severe pneumonia.
- Very rarely a form of encephalitis – inflammation of the brain – can occur, but this is usually in children who have an immune deficiency – for example, those who are being treated for leukaemia. Be on the lookout for neck stiffness, drowsiness and vomiting.

Children on steroid tablets are at special risk of developing a severe form of chickenpox and should see a doctor if they have been in contact with chickenpox. This rule does not apply to children who are taking inhaled steroids for asthma or hay fever.

What else can I do?

Try to persuade your child not to scratch the spots as this may lead to scarring.

If you suspect that your child has any of the above complications, seek medical advice. If you have any ill or elderly friends and family, keep your ill child away from them until the chickenpox has cleared. In particular, keep children away from any woman who is pregnant or potentially pregnant even though she is likely to have already had chickenpox. In the UK, children are not routinely immunised against chickenpox, although an antibody preparation is available for people who have leukaemia or who are having an organ transplant because their immune system is not working properly.

Coeliac disease

What is it?

This is an uncommon disease affecting the part of the bowel called the small intestine. In coeliac disease, the lining of the intestine is very sensitive to a substance called gluten which is commonly found in cereals such as barley, wheat and rye. This sensitivity results in an abnormal immune reaction, damaging the lining of the bowel or small intestine. The small intestine has the important job of absorbing food into the body, so any damage to its inner lining means that food is not absorbed properly.

What action should I take?
Coeliac disease is not easy to diagnose. It can appear at any time after a baby starts taking solids. It can cause weight loss, failure to thrive (see page 29) and even anaemia. Children with coeliac disease rarely become unwell very quickly – instead, they slowly deteriorate. If your child is not thriving take him or her to be assessed by a doctor.

What should I expect?
If your doctor suspects coeliac disease the only way to confirm it is to take samples of the tissue lining the small intestine using a telescope-like instrument. The samples are sent off to the lab and inspected under a microscope, after which it will be very clear if coeliac disease is indicated.

What else can I do?
The treatment for coeliac disease is to exclude foods which contain gluten. Specially prepared gluten-free foods are available on prescription and should be taken only after discussion with a dietitian. A gluten-free diet can be quite restricting and as children grow older, it can be hard to get them to comply with it. Because the gluten-free diet is for life, it is essential that both parents and children understand the nature of the condition and exactly what is in the foods they eat. The Coeliac Society* can offer further advice and support.

Congenital heart disease

What is it?
Congenital heart disease refers to a heart abnormality which is present at birth – in other words, the problem occurred while the baby was developing in the womb. It is usually unclear what caused the defect, although genetic abnormalities can be responsible, as can exposure to viral infections such as rubella in pregnancy (see Chapter 1). There are a huge number of different congenital

abnormalities – some serious and life-threatening, others less significant.

One of the most common abnormalities is the hole in the heart, consisting of a gap, often between the two big pumping chambers of the heart, which allows blood from the left side of the heart to mix with that from the right side of the heart; a big gap may lead to heart failure. Smaller holes in the heart can also be present and may cause no problem, very often closing by themselves as the child gets older. Larger holes which are overloading the heart and causing it to fail may need surgery. If this is the only defect the outlook is usually excellent and you can expect the child to lead a normal life.

Endocarditis is also a risk. This is a potentially nasty infectious condition of the tissue lining the heart, and children with congenital heart disease are at increased risk of developing it. The areas of the body at highest risk are those which are exposed to turbulent blood flow. When bacteria enter the bloodstream, they can colonise the parts of the heart exposed to the abnormal blood flow and cause an infection and a severe illness called bacterial endocarditis.

What action should I take?

Very often the problem will be picked up early, usually at birth, and a specialist will be involved from an early stage. If this is the case, there is little need to do anything. Some of these defects can be quite complex but it is important to try to understand what is going on. Keep asking the specialist, your GP and the health visitor to explain the situation until you understand.

One of the more common causes of bacteria entering the bloodstream is a dental procedure. If your child is at risk of endocarditis he or she should have antibiotics when any dental treatment is given, including fillings, extractions or scaling. The same principle applies to any invasive medical or surgical procedure.

What should I expect?

This really depends on the exact nature of the heart problem and how it was picked up. Some babies and children can be quite unwell, while others have no symptoms and the defect is discovered only during a routine examination. Some affected children and babies will not gain weight properly (see page 29 for more on failure to thrive), while babies with a significant abnormality may be slow feeders and may not have the energy or breath to finish a feed. Some heart defects can cause a bluish tinge on the lips – the 'blue baby' effect. This is because the blood is not all flowing through the lungs so it does not get replenished with oxygen.

When an abnormality is suspected, tests are carried out to try to understand its nature and effects. These tests often include a heart tracing, a chest x-ray and a scan of the heart. The scan will usually be similar to the ultrasound scan performed on pregnant women. These tests do not involve any needles, pain or discomfort and are quite safe. Sometimes, if more information is needed, particularly if it is a complex defect, dye may be injected into the heart via one of the arteries. An x-ray can then be done to outline the chambers of the heart and the pattern of the arteries leading off the heart.

The outlook will obviously depend on the extent of the underlying heart problem but in most cases a solution will be found. If surgery is needed, the vast majority of children do very well. Most children with heart defects, even if they have not needed surgery, will be seen regularly by a specialist called a paediatric cardiologist. These follow-ups can take place over many years and will involve trips to the clinic and possibly repeated tests. Occasionally, more severely affected children will have their care transferred to an adult cardiologist when they are older.

What else can I do?

It is important to make sure that your child has regular follow-up appointments at the clinic. If you move, register with a new GP straight away and get your child referred to an appropriate specialist. On the other hand, try not to be over-protective. Unless you have been told otherwise, your child can lead a normal active life, playing all the same games and sports as his or her friends. If you are in any doubt about this and feel you should be putting limits on your child's activities, check with the specialist.

Be clear about the risks of endocarditis. Make sure you understand whether your child is at risk, what the implications might be and what precautions to take.

Conjunctivitis

What is it?

Conjunctivitis is inflammation of the conjunctiva, the normally transparent thin membrane which lines the front surface of the eyes. It is one of the most common eye diseases and fortunately it either gets better by itself or responds well to treatment. Viral or bacterial infections are the main causes, but allergies such as hay fever can also cause conjunctivitis, as can exposure to smoky atmospheres.

The symptoms of conjunctivitis are fairly obvious: the eyes become red and inflamed and, if the condition is caused by bacteria, a yellow sticky discharge often appears on the eyes and the lids. It is quite common for the eyelids to be gummed together by the sticky secretions, particularly first thing in the morning. Often both eyes are affected but if conjunctivitis starts in one eye the other eye can quickly become affected.

In conjunctivitis caused by an allergy the eyelids can become swollen and itchy and there is also a discharge, although it is usually clear. Often a child with allergic conjunctivitis suffers from hay fever or has a history of allergies. A watery discharge also occurs in conjunctivitis of viral origin.

What action should I take?

For a newborn baby, it is essential to contact the doctor or midwife as soon as possible. If you are still in hospital or receiving postnatal care and neither the doctor nor the midwife has mentioned the redness and inflammation, bring it to their attention. The baby may have picked up some nasty bugs from the birth canal during delivery. If so, these would need to be identified and treated quickly.

In an older child the diagnosis is often very obvious, especially when both eyes are sticky. Take the child to the doctor to establish whether it is conjunctivitis and whether treatment is required to clear it up quickly. Some nurseries or playgroups will not take children with conjunctivitis because it is easily transmissible to other children; they have different policies about how soon they will take children back after treatment has been started.

What should I expect?

Bacterial conjunctivitis is relatively easy to treat and involves the use of antibiotic eye drops or ointment being applied to the eye. Children and babies may not co-operate over this and often the medication seems to go everywhere. However, even a small amount which hits the target may be sufficient. The problem should be resolved very quickly once the treatment is started.

No specific treatment exists for most types of viral conjunctivitis although your GP may prescribe antibiotic eye drops to prevent a bacterial infection superimposing itself on top of the viral infection. Often viral conjunctivitis clears up within a week or so without any treatment, but if it is still present after a week take your child back to the doctor for another check because there are other more serious causes of red eyes. When treatment fails it does not necessarily mean another course of ointment or drops: many serious eye conditions have initially been misdiagnosed as conjunctivitis.

If the problem is allergic conjunctivitis there is no risk of infection but anti-allergy eye drops may be needed to provide relief from the symptoms.

What else can I do?

Regularly bathe the affected eye (or eyes) with cotton wool that has been immersed in lukewarm water. Always use a separate piece of cotton wool for each eye to avoid spreading infection. Wash your hands thoroughly before and after to avoid spreading the infection. In addition, make sure that nobody shares towels or flannels with the affected person – otherwise the infection may spread rapidly though the whole family.

Constipation

What is it?

Constipation is a common childhood condition which causes a lot of concern among parents, but it is not always easy to define exactly what it is. So far as frequency of bowel movements is concerned, there is a wide range of what is normal. Some children pass faeces up to three or four times a day while others do so perhaps only once every three days. Both patterns would be considered normal so long as the routine does not change much.

A more practical way to look at constipation is to think of it as an unusual delay in emptying the bowels. This causes problems if the lower bowel becomes blocked by hard, bulky faecal material. Temporary changes in bowel habit can be brought about by a mild illness or a change in diet. An acute illness resulting in a fever, dehydration and reduced food intake can cause constipation. All these events conspire to reduce the water content of the bowel material and produce hard faeces. This in turn makes it harder to evacuate the bowels and leads to constipation.

Another fairly common cause is a break in the skin around the entrance to the back passage. This is called an anal fissure and it makes passing a bowel motion painful and uncomfortable, so it tends to lead to constipation. Other causes may be poor toilet facilities at school or nursery, which can deter children from emptying their bowels when they need to, or a behavioural problem. For example, children worried about the routines of toilet training may prolong their need to pass a bowel motion.

What action should I take?

It is important to identify the problem correctly in the first place, and that may not be as easy as it seems; the thing to watch out for is a recent change of bowel habit. Paradoxically, constipation may actually present itself as diarrhoea because if the bowel is partially blocked, new material being produced above the blockage may seep out, giving the impression of diarrhoea.

There is no need to rush to the doctor unless your child has failed to pass any faeces for perhaps four days. Don't use laxatives unless a doctor advises you to do so. Constipation can often be sorted out by increasing the number of drinks and the amount of fibre (vegetables, fruit and cereals) in your child's diet. If this does not solve the problem take him or her to the doctor. If your child experiences pain on passing a bowel motion you should also see the doctor about that.

What should I expect?

If you do decide to take your child to the doctor it is unlikely that any tests will be needed. Occasionally an x-ray may be taken which may show a bowel loaded with faecal matter. Your doctor is likely to reinforce the advice to have plenty of fluids and a diet rich in fibre. If the child has an anal fissure the GP may also prescribe a short course of laxatives which will soften the bowel motions and make passing them less painful. The doctor may also prescribe a short course of laxatives to re-establish the normal bowel routine. Once this has happened the laxatives should be stopped. It is very rare for a child to need an enema or a suppository.

What else can I do?

If your child is feverish and has become dehydrated, this may be the cause of the constipation, in which case you may need to treat the cause of the fever (see page 193). If you think there might be a behavioural element to the constipation, watch your child more carefully. Check to see that he or she is not frightened of going to the toilet. If toilet training is proving difficult, try to avoid being confrontational about it. Parents need to be encouraging when their children pass a bowel motion and avoid chiding them if they become constipated again. You could consider using the star reward system as described in the section on bedwetting (page 79).

Convulsions

See **epilepsy**, page 187; **febrile convulsions**, page 31.

Coughing

See **asthma**, page 151; **bronchiolitis**, page 28; **bronchitis**, page 230; **cystic fibrosis**, page 170; **measles**, page 216; **respiratory tract infection**, page 229; **whooping cough**, page 248.

Croup

What is it?

Croup is an inflammation of the big airway in the neck – the windpipe – and the net result is a partial blockage of the windpipe. The most likely cause is an infection; numerous different types of viruses can produce this reaction. The infection is usually spread by inhaling infected droplets or by direct contact with infected secretions such as a runny nose. Typically, it starts with the symptoms of a common cold but after a couple of days or so the child starts breathing noisily as the result of the partially blocked airway.

What action should I take?

The breathing is noisy, which can be alarming in itself, but what you need to monitor is how difficult your child is finding it to breathe. In severe cases he or she can be in obvious distress with fast laboured breathing – contact your GP at once or go to the nearest accident and emergency department. Croup is often worse at night but this should not deter you from seeking urgent medical advice.

In less serious cases, parents are often recommended to 'steam' the room. Even though many doctors think this is an ineffective treatment, placing the child in a warm steamy atmosphere seems to be quite safe. Take your child into the bathroom and turn on the hot water taps, making sure he or she is kept clear of direct contact with the taps and water.

What should I expect?

The noisy breathing that comes with croup – called stridor – can be quite alarming to both parents and children. The child may also have a hoarse voice which reflects the inflammation in the voice box.

What else can I do?

Feverish children should be cooled down with a tepid sponge and, if necessary, can be given paracetamol syrup. Follow carefully the dosage and frequency regime appropriate for your child's age. Children with croup may become dehydrated so make sure they are drinking lots of fluids.

WHAT TO DO IN AN EMERGENCY

If your child is having obvious breathing difficulties, get medical advice immediately. Speak to a doctor on the telephone and either arrange an urgent home visit or take the child straight to the surgery or the nearest accident and emergency department. Do not try to inspect your child's throat in case the cause turns out to be epiglottitis (page 186).

Cystic fibrosis

What is it?

Cystic fibrosis (CF) is a genetically inherited disease, primarily affecting the lungs and guts. In affected children, the fluid that lubricates the airways in the lungs is abnormally sticky, which means that bacteria entering the lungs cannot be removed efficiently. Eventually children with cystic fibrosis develop a long-standing chest infection. In addition, sticky fluid in the gut and glands prevents proper absorption of food, especially fat, so that normal growth is severely inhibited. Children with CF need daily chest physiotherapy to help move the sticky fluid in the lungs from the small to the large airways so that it can be coughed up or spat out. This clears the airways and helps the child breathe more easily.

CF most obviously affects the lungs and the bowel. It leads to recurrent chest infections and, if untreated, the body is unable to absorb fat, resulting in very smelly, greasy stools. But CF can also affect many other body parts and children may suffer from short-term joint pains, non-cancerous growths in the nostrils called polyps, skin rashes, diabetes and liver problems.

Although women with cystic fibrosis themselves can have children, most, if not all, men with CF are sterile. The parents of affected children are usually carriers of CF. This means they have a normal gene on one chromosome number seven and a CF gene on the other. The normal gene is dominant and the parents themselves have no symptoms of CF. In every pregnancy where both parents are carriers there is a one in four chance that the baby will have CF. The affected child inherits a mutant CF gene from both parents. If a woman with CF has a child she will always pass on a CF gene, but a child who has CF will have inherited a CF gene from a carrier father.

The average life expectancy for today's children who have cystic fibrosis is about 40 years so the issue of male sterility needs to be discussed sensitively with boys at a suitable time, usually in their early teens.

Intensive research into gene therapy is expected to produce a cure within the next decade.

What action should I take?

Simple blood or mouthwash sample tests can be done to check

whether or not you carry the CF gene. You should have this done if there is a history of CF in your family. If both you and your partner test positive you will be advised on the various options open to you in any pregnancy. These include testing the baby for CF about 12 weeks into the pregnancy. If the result is positive you can decide whether or not to proceed with the pregnancy.

Children with CF should have a general outpatient review at least every two months by a paediatrician with a special interest in the disease. At least once a year they should go to a major CF centre for a comprehensive clinical review, when they will see a specialist dietitian, physiotherapist and doctor. Your child must see all these people because attention to nutrition and chest physiotherapy are as important as the various medicines that will be prescribed. Many children will receive all their care in the centre, while others may prefer to be looked after in their local hospital with only occasional visits to the CF centre.

DAILY TREATMENT REGIMEN FOR CHILDREN WITH CYSTIC FIBROSIS

The best possible care for a child with cystic fibrosis involves daily treatment at home and includes:

- chest physiotherapy
- antibiotics
- high-energy dietary supplements
- added vitamins
- capsules taken with food to help the gut absorb dietary fat.

Having a child with CF can be stressful for the whole family but it is important both to avoid being overprotective and to make time for family activities. It will help if you talk freely about CF with each other. This will help brothers and sisters to understand why their sibling with CF has special needs and receives more attention. They may need reassurance that they will not develop CF themselves. You should ask your doctor to do a simple diagnostic test for CF on your other children. At a suitable age, usually in their late teens, they can have genetic screening to see whether they are carriers.

What should I expect?

Several hospitals screen all newborn babies for CF using a blood test. Early diagnosis allows early treatment. CF can otherwise become apparent in several ways:

- bowel obstruction at birth
- failure to gain weight
- recurrent chest infections
- very offensive, fatty stools.

Early diagnosis and optimal care will usually allow normal growth and development, and normal childhood activities with full participation in school and sport. At the first suggestion that any of the symptoms may be getting worse – for example, coughing, lethargy, loss of appetite or weight loss – the paediatrician will prescribe some extra treatment. This may be antibiotic tablets or medicine, but treatment with an antibiotic drip or injections may be necessary. This is usually done in hospital but parents can be taught to do it themselves at home.

Apart from the intrusion of the various treatments, most children with CF will have a normal early childhood. There will be some, however, who deteriorate despite the very best care. They will have increasing breathing difficulties but only very rarely need supplementary oxygen or referral for a possible lung transplant.

What else can I do?

Carry out the chest physiotherapy every day at home, encourage your child to exercise and see a CF specialist at least once a year. You should also see your doctor every time your child has a cold, increased coughing, or a raised temperature.

Deafness

What is it?

Deafness is a symptom with numerous possible causes. Some babies are born with it while others develop it as a result of an illness.

The ear relies on two different mechanisms to bring sound to the brain. The sound waves entering the ear cause the eardrum and the bones behind it to vibrate. This vibration is translated into nerve impulses which are then communicated to the brain.

Hearing therefore has a mechanical element – the conduction of sound – and an electrical element – nerve transmission.

Disorders affecting the mechanical element are called conductive deafness; those affecting the electrical part are called sensorineural deafness. The latter can be present at birth, as part of an inherited disorder or caused by an infection during pregnancy. Cytomegalovirus, toxoplasmosis and rubella can all cause deafness (see Chapter 1). But the damage is not always done while the baby is developing in the womb. Sensorineural deafness is one of the complications of bacterial meningitis, for example. It can also be caused by severe jaundice during the period shortly after birth, but this is less common nowadays as jaundice is usually dealt with so promptly.

Conductive deafness is more common and tends to affect older children. A common cause is glue ear (page 199): sticky fluid or 'glue' accumulates in the middle ear and stops the ear bones and ear drum vibrating normally. Another significant cause of conductive deafness is the accumulation of wax, which is produced by glands lining the skin of the ear canal. The role of the wax role is to gather up dust and skin debris in the ear canal and then extrude it. But an accumulation of wax can cause hearing loss simply by blocking the ear canal and making it harder for sound waves to penetrate. Other causes of conductive deafness include a perforated ear drum – the ear drum literally has a hole in it and fails to vibrate properly – which can be the result of injury or infection.

What action should I take?
Babies can hear from an early stage and the first thing is to be aware of the development of a baby's hearing.

HEARING MILESTONES

- Just after birth babies open their eyes or blink in response to a loud noise.
- At four months babies should recognise and respond to a carer's voice even when he or she is not in the line of vision.
- At one year babies may start to utter a few words such as 'mamma' and 'dada'.

It is critical that any hearing deficit is picked up promptly, because impaired hearing will have a catastrophic effect on the development of speech. Although babies undergo a routine hearing test at 7-9 months, don't wait until then if you have any doubts about your baby's hearing.

In older children, ear infections and glue ear account for many hearing problems. Ear infections usually cause symptoms like earache but the symptoms of glue ear may be more insidious, as it is rarely painful. Children with glue ear fail to pick up on conversation and may be falsely accused of inattention at both school and at home. They can end up being labelled as slow learners unless the problem is correctly identified, so it is essential that parents are on the lookout for potential hearing problems. If you are in any doubt, get help.

What should I expect?

All babies and children should have their ears examined if the parents suspect a problem. The GP will look at the internal mechanism of the ear with an otoscope. This is a viewing instrument with a bright light source which is placed in the ear canal. The GP uses it to look at the external ear canal, the amount of wax present, the ear drum and parts of the bones in the middle ear. But the otoscope cannot be used to see the nerve mechanism of the inner ear and sometimes viewing may be incomplete if lots of wax is present.

Older children are relatively easy to assess by simple hearing tests, but younger children and babies are less likely to co-operate so more sophisticated tests are needed – tests which measure the effect a sound makes on the brain, for example.

Problems like excess wax, ear infections and glue ear will need to be treated with syringing, antibiotics, and possibly surgery in the case of glue ear. If babies and children have any significant hearing loss which cannot be reversed, it is important to amplify any sound that can be heard – this often means using a hearing aid. These may not be pleasing, cosmetically speaking, but are a small price to pay for maximising hearing potential. Unless a child has other problems, most with partial hearing loss will attend normal schools. Only those with profound hearing loss will be assessed as having special educational needs. If deafness can be picked up from an early age – the earlier the better – the child stands a good chance of developing understandable speech.

What else can I do?

After the problem has been picked up, it is essential to make the most of your child's hearing potential. Speak directly and clearly. Slightly deaf children need to see your lips move and witness the changes in your facial expression. Always try to make sure that your child has fully understood you. Discuss the problem with teachers and explain that your child has special needs in this respect. If you don't, the teachers may wrongly assume that any inattention is due to laziness. A simple solution may be to sit the child at the front of the class in the optimum position to see the teacher's lips and face.

Children who are more severely affected may need to learn sign language – as will their parents. All parents of children with significant hearing loss should try to understand and sympathise with the frustration that comes from experiencing communication problems.

Diabetes

What is it?

Diabetes is a condition in which the body fails to produce enough insulin to control the amount of glucose – sugar in the blood. Every cell in the body requires glucose for energy to carry out the body's processes. Glucose circulates in the bloodstream once it has been absorbed from the digestive system. The level of glucose in the blood is normally carefully controlled by the hormone insulin, which is produced in the pancreas, an organ situated near the stomach.

There are two main types of diabetes – insulin-dependent (type 1) and non-insulin-dependent (type 2). Type 2 diabetes affects people from their middle age onwards so is not discussed here. Type 1 diabetes is the form which affects children. It is rare before the age of one, but by the age of ten years about 1 in 900 children will have been affected.

In diabetes, insufficient insulin is produced because of damage to the cells of the pancreas. Without enough insulin, glucose cannot enter the body's cells, so the level of glucose in the bloodstream rises. As this happens, glucose spills out into the urine via the kidneys, taking water with it and leaving the body dehydrated.

The exact cause of insulin failure is not known, but it is thought to be due to a combination of inherited, genetic and environmental factors. The environmental factors have yet to be identified, but possible candidates include viral infections.

Diabetes usually starts with marked tiredness, thirst, weight loss and needing to go to the toilet a lot because of excessive urine production. It may first become apparent as a return to bedwetting in a previously dry child. If it is left untreated, these symptoms may lead to drowsiness and even coma.

What action should I take?

If you think your child has the symptoms described above take him or her to see your GP. Take a fresh sample of urine with you in a clean bottle. A simple test can be done there and then to check if there is any glucose in the urine: the doctor simply puts a chemically sensitive stick into the sample. If glucose is present in the urine, the exact level of glucose in the blood will have to be measured, so your child will need to have a blood sample taken for testing.

What should I expect?

If your child does have diabetes he or she will most likely be admitted to hospital for immediate investigation and treatment. If your child is dehydrated, fluids will be given through a drip into a vein. Insulin is given as a series of injections to bring the blood glucose level down; the diabetes is usually stabilised over a period of 24–48 hours.

Once the glucose level is stable you and the diabetes team can start planning the long-term management of the diabetes. A dietitian will help you to adapt your child's eating habits and food choices. A regular insulin dosage will be calculated to maintain the blood glucose at the correct level. The insulin has to be given by injection, often twice and sometimes more, every day.

The blood glucose level is monitored by a finger prick test in which a small blob of blood is placed on a plastic strip which changes colour depending on the amount of glucose present. To start with this has to be done regularly throughout the day, but as time goes on it may have to be done less frequently.

Both you and your child will be taught about diet and diabetes control and shown how to give the injections. Your child will need to go for regular check-ups with the GP and the diabetes clinic at the hospital.

Researchers are currently looking at alternatives to daily injections such as nasal sprays. Ways of transplanting healthy pancreatic tissue into the body are also being tested.

HYPOS

The level of glucose in the blood depends on the amount of insulin given each day, balanced against the amount of food eaten and exercise taken. If for any reason less food than usual is consumed, for example if your child misses a meal, or if more exercise than usual is taken, it is possible for the blood glucose level to drop too far. This is known as a hypoglycaemic attack or 'hypo'. The early signs are dizziness, slow responses, going pale and possibly collapsing.

In the early stages a hypo can be averted by giving sugar in the form of a sugary sweet or a drink such as Lucozade or Ribena or even milk with added sugar. However, a hypo collapse with a loss of consciousness can be treated only by an injection. Sometimes parents or carers are shown how to give the antidote injection, but if this is not immediately available you need to call your doctor immediately or make your own way to the accident and emergency department at the hospital.

What else can I do?

- Learn as much about diabetes as you can, from your hospital diabetes clinic, your GP and the specialist diabetes nurse.
- Contact the British Diabetic Association★ for more information.
- Help your child to keep the diabetes under control. This will minimise long-term complications such as eye disease, heart disease and kidney disease.
- Discuss the problems with friends, family and teachers, and be especially clear about hypos and dietary restrictions. Have a plan of action for the treatment of hypos and make sure everyone around the child understands what to look out for and what to do.

Diarrhoea

See **constipation**, page 166; **gastroenteritis**, page 195; **toddler's diarrhoea**, page 242.

Diphtheria

What is it?

Diphtheria is a bacterial infection spread by personal contact, with humans the only source of infection. Before World War II and the introduction of mass immunisation it was the major cause of death in 4-10-year-olds in England and Wales, and the second most common cause of death in 3-4-year-olds, with 50,000 cases per year. In 1942 there were 2,500 deaths from diphtheria. Mass immunisation had a dramatic effect: by 1950 there were fewer than 1,000 cases and 49 deaths, and in 1965 there were 25 cases and no deaths. Diphtheria is now exceedingly rare in the UK and most doctors will not have seen a case. However, it is still common in countries with poor hygiene and unimmunised people are still at risk, as shown by a recent epidemic in the former Soviet Union. Increasing world travel makes it a risk for everyone.

In the most common form of diphtheria, bacteria multiply on the tissues at the back of the throat. A local and severe inflammatory reaction can produce a thick membrane which obstructs breathing. The infection in fact derives its name from the Greek 'diphthera', meaning a piece of hide or membrane. The bacteria also releases a toxin which damages the nervous system and heart, causing heart failure and paralysis.

What action should I take?

Prevention by immunisation is essential (see Chapter 3) as treatment may not be effective. By the time penicillin is given the bacteria have already released their toxin; penicillin has no effect on the toxin, only on the bug. An antidote – antitoxin – can neutralise the effects of the toxin but by the time this is given it is likely that the toxin has seeded in the tissues where it is inaccessible to any antitoxin in the bloodstream. It is always worth having the antitoxin to try to prevent further serious complications, but it will not reverse the damage already done by the toxin in, for example, the heart or nervous system. Treatment may involve intensive care.

What should I expect?

After an incubation period of three to five days (the time from infection to the appearance of symptoms) the sufferer will be feverish and profoundly tired. The site of infection becomes inflamed and covered by débris and dead tissue. This sticks strongly to the underlying tissues and trying to scrape it off causes pain and bleeding.

The most common form of diphtheria affects the back of the throat and the upper airways that lead down to the lung. Initially the child will be listless and may complain of a sore throat, but won't be noticeably ill for maybe two days. The developing membrane at the back of the throat, together with swollen neck glands, can seriously interfere with breathing. Usually the grey-yellow membrane covers most of both tonsils. In more severe infections the membrane spreads forwards along the palate as far as the front teeth or backwards down the throat.

Because of the threat to life the surgeons may perform a tracheotomy – an operation in which a tube is passed through the front of the neck and into the windpipe below the level of the obstructing membrane. The child will be able to breathe through this tube until the swelling subsides and the membrane shrinks. Other routine treatment includes penicillin drip or injections, antitoxin injections and general help with pain relief and feeding.

Some children just have nasal diphtheria, which appears as a discharge that may be anything from thin and bloodstained to thick and full of pus. These children do not become severely ill themselves but they are very infectious because there are huge numbers of diphtheria bacteria in the discharge. Other sites of infection are the eyes and any areas of broken skin.

The toxin released by the diphtheria bacteria makes the heart muscle flabby and affects the parts of the heart that control the rhythmic beating, so that the heart cannot pump blood around the body properly and may develop a dangerous, abnormal beat. If children recover from the initial attack of diphtheria, they can still die of heart failure in convalescence because when it heals, the damaged heart muscle is replaced with tough fibrous scars and the scarred heart just cannot work properly.

The damage to the nervous system in diphtheria follows a typical pattern. In the third week the palate – the roof of the mouth –

cannot move, so children cannot speak or swallow properly. Around the same time the muscles that control eye movement are affected, resulting in blurred vision. In severe diphtheria, in about the sixth or seventh week, paralysis of the relevant muscles results in further difficulties with swallowing and loss of voice. At the same time paralysis of the muscles used for breathing can be fatal. However, if children survive, they recover fully with no lasting paralysis.

The liver, spleen and kidneys can be damaged by the knock-on effects of severe illness, and abnormalities in the blood-clotting system may result in bleeding. Your child may need to be admitted to an intensive care unit for these complications to be treated.

What else can I do?
Nothing. The best treatment is prevention by immunisation.

Down's Syndrome

What is it?
One of the better-known genetic defects (page 198), this condition – which used to be called 'mongolism' – affects roughly 1 in 700 babies and can occur in the children of all ethnic groups. One of the characteristics of this condition is that it tends to affect babies born to older women. Once a woman reaches the age of 40, the chance of having a Down's Syndrome baby is about one in 100, but younger mothers can also give birth to these babies. The age of the father seems to be irrelevant to the risk of developing Down's. The underlying abnormality is the presence of an extra chromosome – number 21; the condition is also called trisomy 21.

At birth, it may not always be easy to recognise Down's Syndrome babies by looking at their faces, but they are markedly floppy and as they get older the usual characteristics become more obvious. Babies and young children with Down's Syndrome often have protruding tongues and their eyes tend to slope upwards. They are also short and have learning disabilities. Many are born with heart disease and some have bowel abnormalities. As they grow older they show a predisposition to develop certain medical conditions and as a group have an above-average incidence of both leukaemia and dementia. Despite these multiple problems, however, many go on to lead a fairly independent life. Children affected by this condition tend to be affectionate and happy.

What action should I take?

One aspect of antenatal care is screening for diseases in the developing foetus. A simple blood test is offered to all pregnant women, especially older women and those who have previously had a child affected with Down's Syndrome, and if the results suggest a higher than normal risk of the condition, the woman may be offered a further test such as amniocentesis. The amniocentesis test involves taking a sample of the amniotic fluid which surrounds the growing foetus in the womb, while an alternative – chorionic villus sampling – involves taking a sample of tissue from the growing placenta. Both these tests carry a risk of miscarriage and may possibly harm the baby, so it is important to be have a full discussion about the pros and cons before you agree to go ahead (see Chapter 1).

If you have a child with Down's Syndrome, find out as much as possible about the condition. To start with, many parents find it difficult to come terms with both the diagnosis and the outlook for their child. Practical help and advice is available from the Down's Syndrome Association.★

What should I expect?

The diagnosis is likely to be confirmed by a blood test, which reveals the abnormalities in the chromosomes. Once this is confirmed, many parents will be offered genetic counselling. If you are not offered this service ask about it. It is possible that any children you have in the future may at increased risk of developing the same condition.

Once the diagnosis is confirmed, tests will probably be done to look for other abnormalities. For example, babies with Down's Syndrome are usually routinely tested for heart abnormalities. The outlook for those with heart problems has greatly improved over the last few years with the advent of modern effective treatments such as heart surgery. Even so, some Down's babies may not survive childhood because they have severe, untreatable congenital heart disease.

What else can I do?

You can be alert to the special risks which face children with Down's Syndrome. For example, they tend to suffer from lax joints, and the vital neck joints which protect the spinal cord may be weak, increasing the risk of dislocating the neck. This may mean limiting their sporting activities if such a weakness is found. They also tend to have more frequent chest infections and may be prone to an under-active thyroid gland which makes them slow down. This can be easily assessed with a blood test and then treated if necessary.

One of the major problems for babies and children with Down's Syndrome is the delay in their development, but with a lot of stimulation and skilled help their potential can be maximised. This means parents working in conjunction with the various agencies who have something to offer the child, including educational experts, occupational therapists and speech therapists. Your GP should be able to refer you to the appropriate sources.

In the early 1990s the practice of giving Down's Syndrome children high-dose vitamins became quite common, but it has been found to have no beneficial effect on their development and should not be followed. Cranial osteopathy is frequently used but no formal evidence of its benefits has been recorded.

Ear infection

What is it?

Infection can occur in both the external ear canal – otitis externa – or in the middle ear – otitis media. The two types of infection have different causes, symptoms and treatment.

Otitis media

This is by far the most common ear infection in childhood. The middle ear is an air- filled space between the ear drum – the tympanic membrane – and the inner part of the ear. Sounds are transmitted across this space by three tiny bones known as the ossicles. The middle ear is connected to the back of the nose by a canal called the Eustachian tube, one for each ear. Air passes in and out through the tube in order to equalise pressure in the middle ear.

The Eustachian tubes can become blocked, usually as a result of a cold or an allergy such as hay fever. Fluid – often called catarrh –

can build up in the middle ear, causing some hearing loss, often with popping sounds in the ear. The fluid can then become infected by viruses or bacteria, causing the unpleasant symptoms of acute otitis media. An older child will complain of earache, whereas a younger child may simply pull at the affected ear. The child may have a cough, cold or sore throat at the same time, and may be feverish and restless, or scream, vomit or refuse to eat. The ear drum may perforate under the pressure from the fluid, producing a yellow or bloodstained discharge from the ear. If this happens overnight, there may be a stain on the child's pillow. Often the earache improves once the ear drum has perforated because the drum is no longer under pressure. However, you still need to see a doctor for advice.

Otitis externa
Infection of the external ear canal is less common. In fact, it is an infection of the skin of the ear canal, caused by viruses, bacteria or fungi. This area of skin becomes red, weepy or crusty. It is more common in children who suffer from eczema, although it can be caused by a foreign body in the ear canal, such as a bead, which leads to irritation and infection. If you suspect otitis externa, take your child to the doctor, who will examine the ear with a small telescope-like instrument. If the condition is confirmed, the doctor may prescribe a suitable combined antibiotic and steroid eardrop preparation. A similar cream may also be useful for externally inflamed skin.

What action should I take?
If your child is in pain and has a fever you can help by giving paracetamol and sponging with tepid water. You need to see a doctor to get a diagnosis. Acute otitis media is usually treated with an antibiotic medicine, often a penicillin-based one. Your child may also be given a decongestant medicine to try to encourage the fluid to clear.

What should I expect?
After one or two days the child should be brighter, with the pain and fever under control. However, if an antibiotic has been prescribed it is important to complete the course as the fluid can remain in the middle ear for two to three weeks after the infection.

What else can I do?

Ear infections are most common in children aged two to seven. Children with cleft palate are also more at risk. Allergies and parental smoking also make ear infections more likely and it may be these issues that need to be addressed. However, as long as ear infections are not neglected, the child should suffer no long-term impairment of hearing.

Eczema

What is it?

Eczema is a skin condition in which areas of skin become inflamed, red, itchy, dry and scaly. They can also crack and become infected, resulting in weeping and bleeding. In children the most common form of eczema is known as atopic eczema. Atopy is the term used to describe a family predisposition to a variety of conditions including allergies, hay fever and asthma as well as eczema. Eczema may also be caused by an allergy to chemicals, in which case it is often referred to as contact dermatitis. Another form of eczema known as seborrhoeic eczema affects oily areas of skin such as the scalp and face.

Atopic eczema affects about 3 per cent of children. It usually starts at any time from the first few weeks of life up to two years of age but it can occur later in childhood or even in adult life. However, 90 per cent of affected children grow out of the condition by the time they are seven. Atopic eczema mainly affects the baby's face and spreads to the scalp, neck and skin creases as the child grows. The most common skin crease areas affected are the front of the elbows and behind the knees. The condition can vary from mild symptoms and episodes of more severe flare-ups.

What action should I take?

In children with a family history of atopy, certain measures may delay or improve the severity of the condition. Breastfeeding up to or beyond six months is associated with a lower incidence of atopic conditions, for example. It may also help to avoid skin irritants such as biological washing powders, scented soaps and shampoos, baby bath or bubble bath. Bathing in water with a minimum of a plain soap is best.

Once eczema has developed treatment starts with emollients (skin moisturisers) which you can buy from your pharmacist. These are usually creams or bath oils which moisturise and protect the skin. They can be applied often and at any time, but a good time is just after a bath. Remember to pat your child dry, rather than giving him or her a vigorous rubbing with a towel, to prevent skin damage and cracking, which can aggravate the eczema. Your health visitor can give you advice about this early treatment in mild cases.

What should I expect?

If you follow this advice you may be able to control eczema and keep your child's skin healthy, but if this treatment fails you will need to see your GP. The doctor will confirm the diagnosis and explain the treatment options. For example, itching can be reduced by antihistamine medicines which may be sedating (for night-time) or non-sedating (for day-time). If there is any infection on top of the eczema (see impetigo, page 210) an antibiotic can be given, usually as a short course for a few days.

The core treatment is emollients plus short courses of a steroid cream or ointment. Steroids are used to treat eczema flare-ups because of their powerful anti-inflammatory action which reduces the redness, soreness and itching in the skin. They have to be applied sparingly, and you will be advised to use the weakest preparation necessary. One of the commonly used mild steroids is hydrocortisone. Steroids are used for a short period only, especially when applied to the face. You should never use anything stronger than 1% hydrocortisone on a child's face unless you are specifically told to by your doctor. The side effects such as skin-thinning that are associated with the long-term use of steroids are not a problem when creams or ointments are used in short courses.

Many different types of non-steroidal eczema creams, including herbal treatments, are available. Oil of evening primrose capsules have been found to help in some cases; these can be bought from your pharmacist or on prescription and can be used for children over one year old. Homeopathy is commonly used to good effect. There has also been recent interest in Chinese herbal medicines, plant-derived medicines available only through hospital specialists; although some success has been reported with these, the active ingredient has not yet been pinpointed and some people have experienced hepatitis – inflammation of the liver – as a side effect.

If flare-ups become frequent or severe, your child may need to see a skin specialist – a dermatologist – as stronger steroids, further tests and treatments may be necessary. Skin infections, particularly the herpes virus, can cause rapid worsening of the eczema.

What else can I do?
It is important to remember that eczema is not a reason to postpone or ignore the call to have a childhood immunisation.

Further information is available from the National Eczema Society.*

Epiglottitis

What is it?
Epiglottitis is a potentially lethal condition, associated with the bacterium *Haemophilus influenzae,* which results from the epiglottis swelling and creating a serious airway obstruction. The epiglottis is a piece of cartilage which guards the entry to the windpipe, so any swelling here severely limits the flow of air to the lungs. Children with epiglottitis tend to be very ill: they have such great difficulty in swallowing that they cannot even swallow their own saliva. They either spit it out or it collects in the mouth. They are often more comfortable sitting upright but their breathing is usually noisy and obviously difficult.

What action should I take?
Epiglottitis is a medical emergency and should be treated with the same urgency as a case of suspected meningitis. Urgent hospital admission is required.

What should I expect?
An anaesthetist will try to pass a tube down the windpipe and preserve a passage for the air to travel to and from the lungs. This means that the child will have to be put on a ventilator, usually for one to three days. Antibiotics are usually given through a drip into a vein. The child should make a rapid recovery.

What else can I do?

You can have your child immunised against *Haemophilus influenzae.* The vaccine is now given as a routine part of the childhood immunisation programme (see Chapter 3).

WHAT TO DO IN AN EMERGENCY

Apart from recognising the seriousness of the symptoms and obtaining urgent medical help, do not try to alter the child's position by lying him down if he prefers to be upright. If you suspect that the problem may be epiglottitis, don't allow anybody who has not got access to immediate and full resuscitation facilities to inspect the throat, as doing so can block the whole airway and make breathing impossible.

Epilepsy

What is it?

Epilepsy involves fits or seizures which are the result of abnormal electrical impulses spreading through the brain and interrupting normal brain activity. In many cases this results in a loss of consciousness, but it is important to realise that many things cause a loss of consciousness in children and epilepsy is not the cause of all blackouts. A child can lose consciousness because of a simple faint – which is more common in older children – or because of breath-holding (see page 86). Epilepsy is diagnosed only when a child has more than one true fit or convulsion.

In three out of four cases there is no known cause for epilepsy. The remaining cases can be put down to one of a number of conditions affecting the brain such as infection, tumours, head injuries, poisoning and genetic disorders.

Sometimes a fit will come out of the blue, while on other occasions a trigger such as a flashing light may be the cause. There are different types of epilepsy, each with a variety of different symptoms.

Grand mal epilepsy

This is the most common form of epilepsy and is called 'tonic clonic' by some doctors. Grand mal epilepsy involves a sudden loss of consciousness with the risk of possible injury from falling. There is a tonic phase in which the child's limbs stiffen, followed by a clonic phase when his or her body and limbs jerk rhythmically. The attack is usually over in a few minutes. During the attack the child may pass urine or faeces and may bite his or her tongue. After the attack the child may remain drowsy for a while: this is called the post-ictal phase.

Focal epilepsy

In this form of epilepsy the child does not usually lose consciousness or fall although twitching or jerking may occur on one side of the face, arm or leg. The attack may finish then, or it can progress into a full-blown grand mal fit.

Temporal lobe epilepsy

The hallmark of this type of epilepsy is the preceding 'aura' – strange hallucinations or sensations which occur just before the fit. These can be visual images, strange sounds such as humming or buzzing, or strange smells, and they often make a child scream in fear. During the seizure there may be odd movements such as fidgeting or lip-smacking. Not surprisingly, young children find it difficult to describe these sensations, so temporal lobe epilepsy is often difficult to diagnose. In fact, it is common for this type of epilepsy to be misdiagnosed as a behavioural problem or even the result of drug abuse.

Petit mal

These are also called 'absence seizures' and usually occur in children aged five to nine. The attack or seizure lasts between five and 20 seconds, during which time the child goes quiet and vacant. Afterwards the child just carries on what he or she was doing as if nothing had happened. This form of epilepsy rarely persists into adult life.

Infantile spasms

Infantile spasms are very rare, but when they do occur they usually start when a baby is three to nine months old. They involve repeated body spasms lasting only a few seconds, often occurring dozens or even hundreds of times a day. There is often an underlying cause – a developmental abnormality such as a brain malformation, birth injury to the brain through lack of oxygen, or infections such as encephalitis. Infantile spasms often cause a deterioration in a child's mental abilities leading to mental handicap.

What action should I take?

If your child has a fit, the important thing is to prevent injury by clearing the surrounding area of any hard objects or furniture. If possible, put your child in the recovery position – see page 266.

Don't attempt to clear the airway by putting your fingers into the child's mouth. Even though you may panic, try to remember what happens during the fit – the sequence of events and the approximate length of time the fit lasts. This description will be vital in helping doctors to diagnose the cause of the attack, especially if your child has had no previous fits or signs of epilepsy.

If the fit continues for more than a few minutes it is best to call for immediate medical help. You can call your GP, but if there is going to be any delay dial 999 and get an ambulance to take you to hospital. Don't drive to hospital yourself because your child may have a fit on the way and get hurt.

Once you are at the hospital, your child can be given drugs to stop the fit. He or she will probably be admitted for observation and investigation. A fit which stops after two or three minutes may not need such immediate help, but your child should still be assessed by your doctor soon afterwards – on the same day – particularly if this is the first time. If your child has regular fits and you are satisfied that he or she has made a quick and full recovery, there may be no need to see a doctor.

What should I expect?

The GP or casualty doctor will listen to your description of what has happened, examine your child for any underlying illnesses, discuss the possible causes and arrange for a referral to a specialist – a paediatrician or a paediatric neurologist.

Assessing a child with possible epilepsy involves taking lots of details from someone who witnessed the fit, followed by a general physical examination of the child, focusing on developmental milestones and looking in particular at the child's physical and mental abilities, such as language development. Investigations such as blood tests, a skull x-ray and a brain scan may be done as well as an electro-encephalogram (EEG). This is a test which measures the patterns of electrical activity in the brain and may give clues to the type of epilepsy or the area of the brain affected.

A single fit may not necessarily need any treatment, but if recurrent epilepsy is confirmed your child may need drug therapy in the form of medicines or tablets. A number of different drugs are available, each tailored to certain types of epilepsy. Older drugs such as phenobarbitone and phenytoin are being used less these days; children are more likely to be prescribed newer drugs with fewer side effects such as carbamazepine and valproate.

Six or seven out of ten children with epilepsy will find that the condition is well controlled if they take just one type of drug. The others may need to take two different types. The drug dosage may be altered as the child gets bigger or if the fits are not adequately controlled. Ideally, no fits should occur once the drug dosage is right but in practice it is not always possible to eliminate them completely. Your child may have to have further blood tests to check the amount of drug in the blood in order to get the dosage right.

Febrile convulsions rarely continue up to the age of 12. Some 95 per cent of children with febrile convulsions will have stopped by the age of six. Six out of ten children with true epilepsy – not just febrile convulsions – will grow out of it. They will be followed up and monitored by either the hospital specialist or family doctor and if they have been free from fits for two to four years, the decision may be taken to withdraw the medicine gradually over a period of 8 weeks if not months, in the hope that the fits do not return.

What else can I do?

Children with epilepsy should be able to enjoy a normal life with no restrictions on their activities. But a responsible adult should go with them when they are cycling on roads or swimming. If your child does have epilepsy you will need to tell friends, family and teachers. Unless they have other brain problems such as brain damage, most children with epilepsy should attend a normal school.

Further information is available from the British Epilepsy Association.★

Facial swelling

See **mumps**, page 223.

Fainting

What is it?

A faint is a loss of consciousness owing to a sudden and temporary fall in blood pressure which reduces the blood supply to the brain. Basically, the heart temporarily stops pumping enough blood to the brain and the person suffers a blackout. It is very unusual for very young children to faint, but it is more likely to occur when a child is tired or ill. Standing up quickly, particularly in a hot environment, can also cause fainting. A child who faints will look pale and have a rapid but weak pulse. The faint usually lasts one to two minutes, during which the child may twitch but will not jerk and thrash around as in an epileptic fit (see page 187).

What action should I take?

If a child looks as if he is about to faint, either sit him down with the head between the knees or lie him down on the floor, with his legs raised if possible. Try to remember the sequence and timing of events in case you need to describe what has happened to a doctor.

After the faint is over and your child feels hot, loosen the clothing and move him somewhere cooler. Medical help is usually necessary only if children have any signs of a developing illness or do not fully recover from the faint – for example, if they remain drowsy.

What should I expect?

Children usually make a rapid recovery after a simple faint and have no after-effects.

What else can I do?

If your child is prone to fainting you can help by taking a few simple preventative measures. Dressing him in loose, cool clothing on hot days, giving him plenty of drinks and teaching him to get up slowly from a bed or chair can help prevent faints.

DIFFERENCES BETWEEN A FIT AND A FAINT

Although these are typical differences, not all these things happen every time and there are different types of fits. Occasionally, it can be difficult to differentiate between a fit and a faint.

Fit	Faint
Minimal warning of one coming	May be a warning phase
Could happen in any environment	Often a hot environment
Stiff body, rhythmic jerking (tonic clonic movements)	Lying still or mild twitching
	Often quick recovery
Slow recovery	Weak pulse
Normal pulse	Typically child goes a very
Can go red and blue in colour	pale colour

Fever

What is it?

Normal body temperature is between 36°C and 37°C. When someone has a fever it simply means that the body temperature is raised above normal.

Temperature is measured with different types of thermometer. The standard mercury thermometer can be used in the mouth or the armpit. It takes a good few minutes for an accurate reading, so some doctors may instead measure the temperature rectally with an appropriate protective cover over the thermometer. Doctors also have high-tech infra-red thermometers which measure the temperature of the ear drum quickly and accurately. Some parents find it easy to use heat-sensitive strip thermometers which are placed on the child's forehead – these give a reasonably accurate indication of a child's temperature.

The vast majority of fevers in children are caused by an infection, usually viruses triggering colds, sore throats and 'flu, or bacteria which cause ear, chest or urine infections. Other causes are arthritis, inflammatory conditions such as colitis, and immunisations. In the case of infections, as the bugs enter the body they release substances into the bloodstream which alter the settings of the body's own thermostat situated at the base of the brain. One obvious sign of this is shivering, because muscles of the body repeatedly contract in order to create extra heat and this makes the body temperature rise.

What action should I take?

The first treatment for a fever is to remove layers of clothing, sponge with tepid water and give paracetamol, which helps to reduce the temperature and acts as a painkiller. An alternative is ibuprofen, which is used in adults as an anti-inflammatory drug, but can also be given to children. Whichever medicine you use, always check the correct dosage for your child's age. Make sure your child has regular drinks as dehydration is a risk, particularly in the very young child. It is not a major problem if he does not eat, but he must drink adequate amounts of fluids. As a general guide, children under a year should have 50–100ml every four hours; children aged one to two years should have 150ml every four hours and children over two years should have 250ml every four hours.

You should also look out for symptoms which will give you a clue about the cause of the fever:

- runny nose, sore throat or earache
- cough, wheeze or croup
- urine infection – mainly in girls – frequent trips to the toilet, tummy ache, blood in urine (which may be pink)
- rash, which could be chickenpox, measles or German measles
- diarrhoea and vomiting
- abdominal pain – in which case appendicitis may be a possibility
- headache, stiff neck, dislike of bright light, drowsiness, vomiting, purple rash – signs of meningitis.

See the index for all these problems.

What should I expect?

A fever will usually respond to the simple measures given above. If it becomes obvious that your child has one of the common childhood illnesses this may be all you need to do. However, certain conditions will need advice and treatment from a doctor, such as earache, severe coughs or abdominal pain. Any fever above 40°C or one which is not settling, particularly in a baby under one year old, needs medical attention. If you suspect a serious condition such as meningitis, get medical help immediately.

What else can I do?

A fever which does not settle or a fever which has no obvious cause needs to be investigated further. Don't be afraid to go back to your doctor again if you are worried. The less common forms of infection such as liver or kidney infections, tuberculosis or malaria may need to be considered. Blood tests, urine tests or a chest x-ray may be done and your child may need to be referred to a paediatrician.

See also: chickenpox (page 160); meningitis (page 219); mumps (page 223).

Fits

See **epilepsy**, page 187; **febrile convulsions**, page 31.

Fragile X Syndrome

What is it?

Fragile X Syndrome has only recently been recognised as a relatively common cause of developmental delay and learning difficulties. It is thought to affect about 1 in 1,000 boys and 1 in 2,500 girls. People with Fragile X Syndrome can have an abnormal appearance: affected boys and men tend to have a big face and ears and, after they attain puberty, they can have large testicles. Some boys may also exhibit some of the behavioural problems seen in autism. The diagnosis is made after a blood test: by examining genetic material doctors can see whether there is an abnormality on the X chromosome, one of the so-called sex chromosomes.

What action should I take?

Although the blood test is relatively simple, this is not an easy condition to diagnose because many of its characteristic features do not appear until after puberty. However, if your child shows signs of abnormal behaviour or learning difficulties you could discuss with your doctor the possibility of this condition and ask if it is worth doing a test to examine the chromosomes.

What should I expect?
If your child is diagnosed as having Fragile X Syndrome you should expect to receive some genetic counselling. The condition itself is untreatable so the important thing is to get help in meeting your child's special needs. This help should include a customised educational programme which will maximise his or her potential.

What else can I do?
As with many genetic conditions a fair amount of exciting research on Fragile X Syndrome is being carried out, so it is worth trying to keep up to date. The condition can be passed on through many generations, so counselling and chromosome tests may be needed to see whether any women in the family are carriers. Further information is available from the Fragile X Society.*

Gastro-enteritis

What is it?
Gastro-enteritis, otherwise known as a tummy upset or a tummy bug, is the name given to diarrhoea and vomiting caused by a bacterial or viral infection of the gut, and is one of the most common childhood illnesses. There are about 500 million cases of gastro-enteritis each year in developing countries where it can be a serious illness causing many deaths. In westernised countries gastro-enteritis usually follows a mild course, although it still accounts for about 20 per cent of outpatient paediatric referrals in the USA. Only the common cold attacks more children.

Gastro-enteritis commonly affects children under two years old, although it can affect people of any age. Bacterial gastro-enteritis can be caught from infected and undercooked food such as meat, poultry and eggs. Children can also be infected by playing with pets, usually puppies, who have a tummy bug themselves. The infection gets on to the children's hands and, if they are not properly washed, into their mouths when they suck their fingers or feed themselves.

Other types of gastro-enteritis can be contracted from contaminated water. Any of these infections may be spread direct from one child to another when they play together, and also when parents touch one child, contaminate their hands, and then touch another child.

What action should I take?

Most episodes of gastro-enteritis are short-lived and need no special treatment. It is most important that your child drinks enough, so that the fluid lost with the diarrhoea and vomiting is replaced. Don't worry if he does not eat very much at the height of the illness – he will probably make up for it as soon as he feels better.

You should consult your doctor if a small baby is involved, because he or she could rapidly lose significant amounts of fluid and become dehydrated. You should also see the doctor if vomiting is severe, if your child has a raised temperature or blood in the diarrhoea, or if your child is showing signs of dehydration (increasing apathy and listlessness, dry skin, dry tongue, sunken eyes and decreased urine output).

What should I expect?

Most children can be treated at home. If there are signs of dehydration your doctor can prescribe a rehydration solution, such as Dioralyte, Electrolade or Rehidrat, which contains a balanced amount of sugar, salt, potassium and other minerals that will maintain the normal amounts in the blood. These can also be bought over the counter at a pharmacy without a prescription. They should not be taken for longer than one day before you start giving normal drinks again. Children with gastro-enteritis do not need to be starved and you don't have to stop breastfeeding. All children with mild to moderate diarrhoea can continue to have their normal drinks, and these should be offered frequently and in small amounts. They can also continue to take solid foods.

Don't be alarmed if your baby passes small amounts of blood in faeces. This is quite common with some bacterial gut infections like salmonella and is just the result of the bug damaging the lining of the gut. You should, however, see your doctor because he or she might want to do some blood tests and send off a sample to the laboratory just as a precaution.

In any case, if the diarrhoea does not settle within a few days, your doctor will send a sample to the laboratory to try to find the cause of the infection. Most episodes are caused by viruses and these do not need any specific treatment. Some bacterial infections do respond to antibiotics, but most will steadily improve over a few days without the need for anything other than making sure the child has enough to drink.

Sometimes babies continue with diarrhoea because the infection has damaged the surface of the gut and they cannot digest milk proteins. This is treated by giving the baby a soya-based or other specially prepared milk which does not irritate the gut. After a few weeks babies will be able to take their usual milk again when their bowels have returned to normal. Because the problem is an intolerance to cow's-milk protein, breastfed babies will suffer from it only if their mothers are drinking milk which is passed into the breastmilk. In this case, the mother should use a milk substitute and calcium supplement for a few weeks.

If your child refuses to drink and is losing a lot of fluid because of persistent vomiting or diarrhoea, hospital admission may be necessary, and a fluid drip containing sugar and salt may be given for a few days. Small drinks will also be given and gradually increased as the acute illness settles.

What else can I do?

Remember to be meticulous with your personal hygiene. Dispose of dirty nappies in plastic bags. Wash your hands carefully after cleaning or handling your child, and before preparing any family meals.

WHAT TO DO IN AN EMERGENCY

Only very rarely do emergencies develop from childhood gastro-enteritis. If your child suddenly becomes very quiet and floppy, develops a high temperature, or seems to be in a lot of pain, call your doctor or take the child to your local accident and emergency department. These signs can reflect significant dehydration, spread of the infection into the bloodstream, or some underlying complication.

Genetic abnormalities

What are they?

Genetic abnormalities result from the genes which are passed down from parent to child. At the centre of most cells of the body is a nucleus, within which lie the chromosomes. Grouped within these chromosomes are genes which contain chemical codes that convey unique information about us: hair colouring, build and predisposition towards illness are just some of the many characteristics contained within them.

Although genetic information is inherited from the parents, it does not always follow that the child's health and development are pre-ordained. Environmental factors such as parental attitudes, lifestyle, exposure to certain concepts and philosophies and environmental hazards such as air pollution and toxins will also greatly influence health and development. It is the interaction of the two variables, genetic and environmental, which makes us unique. It is also this cocktail which will determine our risk of developing diseases. Some diseases or illnesses may be wholly determined by our environment. For example, the chances of being involved in a car accident represent an environmental risk, not a genetic risk. At the other end of the spectrum certain genetic mixes will result in diseases or disorders, such as sickle-cell disease, Down's Syndrome and cystic fibrosis (all covered in this A-Z).

Many diseases involve interactions between genetic and environmental factors. Heart disease, for example, may be partially derived from an environmental risk such as smoking and a genetic risk such as high cholesterol (although this can also have environmental origins, such as a cholesterol-rich diet).

In the last few years, great strides have been made in our understanding of genetically based disorders.

What action should I take?

You may already know that a genetic disease such as cystic fibrosis runs in the family, or that you may be at higher risk of having a genetic disease. For example, older women who are pregnant are at higher risk of carrying a baby with Down's Syndrome. It is possible to screen for Down's Syndrome and other genetic disorders during pregnancy and you can discuss this with your midwife, GP or obstetrician (see Chapter 1).

If you have already had a baby with a genetic abnormality or you think a genetic condition runs in your family, it makes sense to seek expert advice. Ideally this should be done before conception – your GP should be able to refer you to a clinical geneticist.

What else can I do?

When you are looking at your family history get exact details of who suffered from what and what relationship they are to you. Geneticists often draw up a family tree to try to help them identify the risk to you. If a genetic illness runs through the family try to obtain further information about the condition, perhaps from one of the many self-help groups which can provide further information about illnesses or diseases which have a genetic influence. The Patients Association★ maintains a database of self-help groups covering a wide range of conditions, not just genetically derived diseases.

Glandular fever

See **hepatitis and liver disease**, page 204.

Glue ear

What is it?

Glue ear is the name given to a condition in which the fluid built up in the ear becomes thicker and persistent. This may happen if a child suffers from repeated ear infections. About one in 25 children are estimated to develop glue ear at some time. The significance of this condition is that it can affect a child's hearing (see page 172) as the sticky fluid or glue stops the ear bones and ear drum vibrating normally. A child may complain of hearing loss or it may be suspected if a child appears to be inattentive at home or at school.

What action should I take?

If you suspect that your child may have glue ear or a hearing problem, it is important to see your health visitor or doctor. Your child may be sent for a formal hearing test, usually at the hospital.

What should I expect?
If glue ear is confirmed, the doctor may start by recommending treatment with decongestants, although some doctors doubt whether they work. If the problem persists, however, your child might be offered a small operation. This involves a small plastic bobbin-shaped tube called a grommet being stitched into the ear drum. This allows air to circulate freely within the cavity of the middle ear and stops the fluid accumulating. Most grommets work their way out of the ear drum within six months to a year, by which time it is likely that the glue ear will have cleared up, although a few children go on to develop glue ear again once the grommet has come out. It is quite possible to have the grommets replaced by a second operation.

What else can I do?
Monitor your child's hearing and see the doctor if you feel it is getting worse. Some parents have found that homeopathy has helped children with glue ear.

Hand, foot and mouth disease

What is it?
This is a minor infection, mainly affecting children in epidemics and most commonly in the spring months. It is caused by a virus but is not at all related to foot and mouth disease in cattle. The affected child is not usually ill, but develops small blisters which sometimes look like chickenpox blisters, although they appear only on the hands, feet and mouth. In the mouth they can occur on the inside of the cheeks, on the tongue and outside on the lips.

What action should I take?
Hand, foot and mouth disease is a minor condition and there is no specific treatment, so don't worry about it. All you need to do is keep the affected areas clean, to prevent a bacterial infection developing on top. It may be worth a trip to the doctor if only to confirm the diagnosis and reassure you.

What should I expect?
Your child should not become ill, and the spots should clear up in a few days.

What else can I do?

The illness can be passed on to adults as well as children, and teachers and playgroup leaders are often worried about it. You may need to keep your child away from school, nursery or playgroup until the spots have cleared.

Hay fever

What is it?

Hay fever is basically an allergy to pollen, but 'hay fever' is not a good term, as hay is not really the cause of the problem and there is no fever. From the end of March into late summer various trees, plants, grasses and crops release pollen into the atmosphere.

These pollens can provoke an allergic reaction wherever they come into contact with the body's membranes. Normally this sort of reaction is a protective response, but in hay fever it is inappropriate, exaggerated and unwanted.

The characteristic symptoms of hay fever are:

- itchy, watery, swollen eyes
- blocked or runny nose and sneezing
- throat irritation
- wheezing or worsening of asthma.

As most sufferers have nasal symptoms, the term rhinitis is sometimes used instead of hay fever. Seasonal rhinitis describes hay fever, whereas perennial rhinitis describes similar nasal symptoms occurring all year round, in response to other allergens as opposed to just pollens.

What action should I take?

Look out for the symptoms in your child, especially if there is a family history of allergies, asthma, hay fever or eczema. There are things you can do to try to minimise the symptoms by reducing the child's exposure to pollen but in some cases they may be impractical. For example, you can avoid going out into fields on warm, sunny days; keep the house windows closed; dust with a damp cloth; wash everybody's clothes regularly; and make sure the child takes regular baths or showers.

You can also get advice and treatment from your pharmacist or doctor. Each separate symptom can be treated with eye drops, antihistamines, steroid nasal sprays and asthma inhalers. When used in short courses steroids do not have the side effects associated with long-term use.

Hay fever as a whole can be treated with antihistamines in the form of tablets or medicines but often a combination of treatments is necessary. Be prepared to try several different preparations to treat the condition. The older antihistamines used to make people drowsy but the newer ones avoid this problem.

Hay fever sufferers have found certain homeopathic remedies helpful. Avoiding refined sugar and dairy products can sometimes help allergic conditions such as hay fever, asthma and eczema, but remember that dairy products are a very important source of calcium and vitamins for the growing child.

What should I expect?

The severity of hay fever symptoms can vary during the season depending on the weather and the different types of pollen present in the air at any particular time. Treatment is best started as soon as symptoms appear and should continue for a few days after they have settled. Severe or persistent symptoms may require continuous treatment throughout the season. Watching the weather forecasts and pollen counts may serve as warnings of the periods of high risk.

What else can I do?

If your child's hay fever is severe or prolonged the doctor may prescribe a short course of steroid tablets. These are effective in the short term and may help a child if there is an important event such as exam coming up. Steroids have no adverse effects when used in short courses and they are very effective in relieving the misery of hay fever.

Headache

What is it?

A headache is a pain in any part of the head. Headaches may be sharp or dull pains and may be associated with other symptoms such as nausea or flashing lights. Less than one per cent of all headaches are a sign of serious physical problems. This small percentage includes headaches caused by, or occurring after, concussion or injury to the head, meningitis, encephalitis (inflammation of the brain), stroke or brain tumours. In children, most headaches are associated with fevers or general illness. Sometimes headaches can be caused by stress and often no cause is found.

Migraines involve recurrent, severe and usually throbbing headaches, accompanied by nausea, sometimes by impaired vision and often on one side of the head only. A migraine attack can be started by stress.

Simple headaches are usually associated with fevers and infections in the respiratory tract or urinary tract. Headaches that are accompanied by drowsiness, neck stiffness, aversion to light, rashes and vomiting are potentially serious, as these are signs of meningitis (see page 219). A headache linked with double vision or an unsteady gait could indicate a serious problem, since these are symptoms of brain disease.

What action should I take?

In most cases all you need to do is treat the symptoms with paracetamol or ibuprofen preparations specially designed for children. Do not use any aspirin products for children under the age of 12 as there is a danger of causing a serious illness called Reye's Syndrome. If you are in any doubt as to the cause of the headache, get help from your GP. Many parents are afraid that a headache is an underlying sign of a serious disease but in the vast majority of cases there is nothing to worry about.

What should I expect?

Most headaches should either get better themselves or with the use of simple pain killers. If a headache lasts longer than a few days or if other symptoms are present you should take your child to the doctor.

What else can I do?

Try to work out whether there is anything such as stress or anxiety which could be causing your child's headaches. If the headaches keep recurring, take him to see your doctor. Some children may be helped by acupuncture.

Hepatitis and liver disease

What is it?

Hepatitis is a viral infection of the liver and is a major cause of liver disease in children (jaundice in newborn babies is discussed in detail on page 21). The liver is the largest of the body's so-called solid organs (the skin being the largest organ overall). It has many different functions, including storing energy in the form of the carbohydrates, glucose and glycogen; manufacturing important body chemicals such as proteins, fats, cholesterol and hormones; and breaking down and removing harmful substances such as drugs, alcohol and poisons from the bloodstream.

Any condition which upsets the way the liver works can cause:

- loss of appetite, nausea and vomiting, tummy pain and weight loss – because the digestion is affected
- yellow skin (jaundice) – because the level of the chemical bilirubin rises in the bloodstream
- dark urine and pale stools – again because of the increased bilirubin
- abnormal bleeding and bruising – because of problems with blood clotting
- fluid retention and body swelling – because of low protein levels in the blood.

In children, the major cause of liver disease is hepatitis, which is a viral infection of the liver. This is usually hepatitis A, but can be hepatitis B or hepatitis caused by glandular fever. Rarer causes of liver disease include leukaemia, tropical infections and liver tumours.

Hepatitis A

Otherwise known as infectious hepatitis, this is caused by the hepatitis A virus. It is transmitted from one person to another by mouth or through faeces, or contaminated water, milk or seafood. The incubation period – the time between infection and the appearance of symptoms – is about two to four weeks and symptoms exhibited may be tiredness, fever, vomiting and diarrhoea. These so-called prodromal symptoms may be mild or even overlooked in younger children. Almost all children will be better in about six weeks and a full recovery can be expected.

Hepatitis B

Otherwise known as serum hepatitis, this is a more severe illness but is much rarer in children. It is usually transmitted through contact with the blood of an infected person. Blood transfusion used to be a risk, but now all blood in the UK is screened for such viruses and is considered safe. Open wounds, pricks from infected needles and tattooing are possible causes. It is also possible for hepatitis B to be passed from an infected mother to her baby during or shortly after birth. It is not thought to pass across the placenta during pregnancy.

Many people who have had hepatitis B may recover from the illness, but remain carriers of the virus and therefore can remain a silent hazard to other people. Hepatitis B has a longer incubation period than hepatitis A – about one to five months. The symptoms are the same as for hepatitis A but they are often much more severe. Additional symptoms, such as painful joints – arthritis – or itchy rashes, can also occur. A minority of sufferers will go on to have chronic liver disease or become carriers. This in turn can lead in later life to diseases such as cirrhosis of the liver and liver cancer.

Glandular fever

This is another viral infection which causes swelling of the glands, rashes and a sore throat illness often confused with tonsillitis. The spleen and liver may also become involved, causing hepatitis-like symptoms. Glandular fever can produce symptoms of tiredness which can last from a few weeks to a few months. The diagnosis is made by a blood test looking for a particular abnormality.

What action should I take?

Any child who develops jaundice should be seen by a doctor. Blood tests are likely to be done in order to work out which virus is causing the infection. All that is needed is treatment of the main symptoms, so fluids, paracetamol and possibly an anti-sickness medicine can be given.

Children with hepatitis A can usually be looked after at home. Immunisation can be offered, but the main precaution is good hygiene, especially when handling food. Children with hepatitis B may need to be go into hospital, depending on the severity of their symptoms. Family members and close contacts need to be protected and this may mean offering them immunisation against hepatitis B.

What should I expect?

With hepatitis A, full recovery is usual after about six weeks, and no further action is necessary. But hepatitis B sufferers need to have further blood tests to check whether the infection has cleared or if they have become carriers of the disease.

What else can I do?

Immunisation against hepatitis A is available and is advisable when you are travelling to certain areas of the world where the infection is common. It is also important to take basic hygiene precautions in these countries, especially with food and water. Hepatitis B immunisation is recommended mainly for adults in 'at-risk' professions; this includes ambulance crew, doctors, nurses and police. Children are generally immunised only if they have a family member with the condition but are given the hepatitis A jab if necessary for foreign travel.

Hernia

What is it?

A hernia is the protrusion of an organ or part of an organ or other internal structure through the wall of the cavity that normally contains it. Usually this means that part of the intestine is protruding through the abdominal wall because of a defect in the muscles. Hernias may be present at birth (**congenital hernia**), or they can develop over months or years. In children they are generally due to a minor congenital problem with the formation of the abdominal wall. Occasionally, inguinal hernias (see below) are accompanied by a hydrocele, which is an accumulation of fluid around the testicle. They are painless and many disappear by themselves within the first year of life. However, if they persist your child will need to have an operation.

An **inguinal hernia** is one that passes through the abdominal wall in the groin area. In boys, this may lead to a swelling in the scrotal sac as a length of bowel escapes from the abdominal cavity and descends down a canal in the groin.

A **diaphragmatic hernia** is one in which part of the stomach or a loop of the intestine protrudes upwards through an opening in the diaphragm into the chest cavity. This is rare in children, but occurs when there is a defect in the diaphragm muscle which separates the thorax (the chest cavity) from the abdomen. This usually happens while the baby is growing in the womb and it can also mean that the lungs fail to develop properly. You cannot see the hernia but it would be picked up on an antenatal ultrasound scan.

An **umbilical hernia** is one in which the bowel, or the membranous apron overlying it, protrudes through the abdominal wall under the skin near the navel. This is relatively common at birth.

What action should I take?
If you notice any swelling under the skin, protrusion in the abdominal wall or swelling in the scrotum you should take your child to see a doctor.

What should I expect?
Many umbilical hernias resolve on their own and do not need any medical or surgical intervention. However, all inguinal hernias require surgery. This is usually a very simple procedure done under a general anaesthetic. A diaphragmatic hernia is a serious condition which can prove fatal because of its effect on the lungs.

What else can I do?
Once you have been told that your child has a hernia it is important to look for changes. If the swelling can be easily reduced (a medical term meaning that you can gently push the swelling back into the abdominal cavity), then there is no immediate problem. If you cannot reduce the swelling, although you used to be able to, or if it enlarges or changes colour, or if the child is obviously in pain, this could indicate a condition called strangulation. This means that the hernia is blocked from sliding back and that its blood supply may be getting cut off. This is a surgical emergency, and you must talk to your GP urgently or take your child to the nearest accident and emergency department.

Human Immunodeficiency Virus infection (HIV)

What is it?
The human immunodeficiency virus attacks the core of the body's

defence against infection. HIV-positive children become more susceptible not only to the common infections that affect us all, but also to so-called opportunistic bacteria, viruses and fungi that are easily destroyed by an intact immune system.

For children the main sources of HIV infection are:

- an HIV-positive mother who can pass on the virus during pregnancy or delivery (this happens in about 13 out of 100 cases)
- breastfeeding
- transfusions with contaminated blood or blood products (in all developed countries where blood donors are screened for HIV this is no longer a risk)
- needle-stick injuries from dirty needles which have been used by infected intravenous drug abusers and which have not been disposed of safely.

There are no genes involved in HIV infection, so the only risk from an HIV-positive father is that he will infect the mother during unprotected sex.

What action should I take?

Antenatal clinics in the UK do not perform routine blood tests for HIV infection, but it makes sense to request these tests if there is any risk you are HIV-positive. This is important because treatment during pregnancy and in the baby's first weeks of life can significantly reduce the risk of the baby becoming infected.

The risk from needle-stick injuries is small. The virus is fragile and does not live long outside the body. You should, however, clean the wound thoroughly and see your own doctor who will take advice from the local specialist. A drug that can prevent multiplication of the HIV virus may be prescribed. Blood tests will be done for up to three to six months to look for any sign of HIV infection.

What should I expect?

If you are pregnant and you know or discover you are HIV-positive, your obstetrician will discuss with you the risk of your baby becoming infected and the pros and cons of interventions that might reduce this risk. For example, you could take anti-viral drugs in late pregnancy and deliver by caesarean section. These anti-viral drugs will reduce risk of transmission from 13 to 8 per cent, and having a section could halve the risk of transmission. The paediatrician who will look after your baby will also see you during pregnancy and discuss with you how your baby will be treated in the first few weeks of life.

It will be several months before blood tests can rule out or confirm HIV infection in a newborn baby, so your baby may be given anti-viral drugs for the first six weeks. Because opportunistic infections are a major cause of death in the first year, babies at risk of HIV will be given antibiotics to prevent such infections until it is established whether they are HIV-positive or not. They will be reviewed regularly by the paediatrician who will ask parents in detail about the baby's general health, look for any signs of infection, check developmental progress and record gains in weight and length.

All babies with HIV infection are given all the routine childhood immunisations (see Chapter 3), except the BCG vaccine for protection against tuberculosis. The latter contains a bacterium that can itself cause a serious illness in children with a defect in the immune system. For all the other immunisations, the danger from the infections outweighs any risk of giving the vaccines. The immunisations are given in the first few months of life, before the child's immune system is severely damaged by the HIV infection, and while he or she can still respond to the vaccine.

HIV infection in children is different from that in adults. There is a shorter incubation period so that most children become ill within the first few years and up to half die before the age of five. The main problems are:

- recurrent and severe infections
- failure to thrive
- developmental delay
- large liver and spleen
- enlarged glands.

All HIV-positive children must be cared for by a specialist hospital team including a doctor, dietitian and counsellor. The team will advise you about routine problems and will work in conjunction with your family doctor.

What else can I do?

Get your child immunised in the routine way as advised. It is extremely important that children who are HIV-positive are treated promptly and appropriately at the first sign of any infection. You must contact your doctor whenever your child is ill and you must attend for the regular outpatient reviews even if you think your child is completely well. It is essential for the doctor to see you frequently so that any problem that is brewing can be picked up as soon as possible.

Impetigo

What is it?

Impetigo is a skin infection caused by bacteria, an example of which is called *Staphylococcus aureus*. The bacteria get in places where the skin is broken, such as small cuts, scratches or patches of eczema. Impetigo is most common around the nose and mouth. In fact, the bugs can be harboured in the nose and the nasal passages and can act as a source of infection. Impetigo spreads easily to other areas of the body and from one person to another.

What action should I take?

Try to prevent the infection spreading by stopping your child from scratching or picking the infected area – easier said than done. Don't let anyone else use the flannel, towels and cups used by your child either at home or at school. You can wash the spots with warm water to remove the crusts gently, but you usually need to visit the doctor who can prescribe an antibiotic cream or an antibiotic medicine or both, depending on the extent of the impetigo. You must tell your child's teacher and make sure your child understands how important it is not to share food or drinks with anyone.

What should I expect?

Initially, a red patch appears, increases in size, begins to form small blisters and then weeps a yellow fluid. This fluid then dries, forming golden yellow crusts on the skin. Within a few days the affected areas should have stopped spreading and the yellow crusts should no longer be forming. The remaining pink or red patches will then fade over the next week or two.

What else can I do?

If impetigo becomes a recurrent problem, the doctor may look for an underlying skin problem such as eczema or scabies, which involves breaks in the skin surface, so keep a look out for tiny cuts or wounds. If you see any, swab them with a general antiseptic liquid. On very rare occasions repeated episodes of impetigo may indicate a problem with the immune system.

Jaundice

See **hepatitis and liver disease**, page 204; and **jaundice** in newborn babies, page 21.

Leukaemia

What is it?

Leukaemia is a cancer of the blood and the blood-forming tissues in which there is an overproduction of immature white blood cells. There are two forms of leukaemia – acute and chronic. Acute leukaemia is most common in children and in young adults, particularly children between one and five years old. Chronic leukaemia tends to occur in adults.

In the vast majority of cases doctors are unable to establish the exact cause of the problem, but certain factors have been associated with some leukaemias. For example, some genetic defects such as Down's Syndrome may predispose a child to developing leukaemia, and exposure to ionising radiation and certain chemicals (e.g. benzene) is associated with an increased risk of leukaemia.

Whatever the cause, normal blood cells and marrow cells (where blood cells are formed) are transformed into malignant cells. This process appears to start in a single cell which then multiplies, repeating the fault.

What action should I take?

As soon as a GP suspects leukaemia he or she will refer the child immediately to a specialist, but it is very unlikely that parents themselves would suspect leukaemia because the symptoms may be non-specific. In general, the child will be ill and seem anaemic – pale, tired and lethargic. The child may also bruise or bleed easily and may suffer recurrent infections, often of the tonsils. When major organs are affected the symptoms are those of damage to those organs.

What should I expect?

The symptoms of leukaemia are caused by the lack of normal blood cell formation and the infiltration of the organs by the faulty cells. Organ infiltration results in enlargement of the liver, spleen and lymph nodes, and possibly the kidneys and testicles as well. The linings of the brain can also become infiltrated with leukaemic cells and this produces a meningitis-like syndrome. The diagnosis of leukaemia is made on the basis of the child's symptoms plus laboratory tests on blood samples and bone marrow samples.

Intensive drug treatment – chemotherapy – is the main treatment for getting rid of the faulty cells and restoring normal blood cell production in the bone marrow. Drugs are selected according to the sensitivities of specific leukaemias and are usually given in combination. Radiotherapy may be used as well to treat local accumulations of leukaemic cells. Surgery is rarely needed to deal with the leukaemia but may be used to manage some of the complications. Sometimes a child may need a bone marrow transplant from a close relative but this works only when there is a very close match between the donor and the recipient.

What else can I do?

The diagnosis of leukaemia means a radical change both to the child's life and that of the immediate family. Despite this, it is important for all involved to try to lead as normal a life as possible. The treatment, particularly chemotherapy, makes infection more likely because it can damage and hinder the responses of the immune system, so it is vital that children having chemotherapy should be kept well away from other children with viral or infectious illnesses such as chickenpox. Any child with an impaired immune system who may have been exposed to an infectious disease should get advice from a doctor. In the case of chickenpox, for example, an injection of antibodies could be given.

A parent could consider being tested as a possible bone marrow donor. A simple blood test can reveal information about your bone marrow which can be stored in a database and matched with information from someone requiring a bone marrow transplant. This is one method of finding unrelated donors. Write to the Anthony Nolan Bone Marrow Trust★ for more information.

WHAT TO DO IN AN EMERGENCY

What is a minor problem for most children may be an emergency for a child having treatment for leukaemia. For example, a temperature or a rash can be quite dangerous and should be treated as an emergency. Often the hospital unit treating the child will see him or her directly without having to go through the family doctor.

Lice infestation

What is it?

The louse is an insect that lives on, and feeds off, its human host. Lice infestations occur all over the world, with major epidemics during wars and in overcrowded living conditions. In the developed world, head lice can be found in about 9 per cent of children at any one time, in all social classes, and children account for around 60 per cent of all cases.

The body louse and the head louse are very similar, but unlike body lice infestation, **head lice** infestation does not reflect standards of personal hygiene. The lice have no preference for dirty or even long hair. They live close to the scalp and lay their eggs near the hair roots. It is the egg capsules – the nits – that can be seen attached to the hairs. About seven to ten days after they are laid, the eggs hatch, the baby lice feed and grow, and after two to three weeks the now mature adults mate. The female will produce up to 300 eggs over the next three to four weeks before her own death. Spread of the infestation is mostly through close contacts within families. One of the major symptoms is itchiness.

Body lice are caught by close contact with infested people or materials like bedding, clothes or towels. Their eggs look very similar to those of head lice. The adult body lice are about 3-4.5mm (just under half an inch) long. They have three pairs of legs, each with claws for gripping, Although there may be many eggs (nits), there are not usually more than 10 to 20 lice on most infested people.

What action should I take?

Repeated **head lice** infestation is quite common as many family members can be infested simultaneously. The problem is cured and controlled by treating the whole family with lotion and shampoos that kill the lice. The lotions are rubbed into dry hair and the scalp, combed through and allowed to dry naturally; they are washed off 12 hours later. The shampoos are left on for five minutes, rinsed off and the process repeated before combing. The shampooing should be repeated three days later. To remove dead nits, wet the hair with a solution made up with equal volumes of water and vinegar, and comb the hair with a fine-toothed comb that has itself been dipped in vinegar. Some authorities recommend that combs and hairbrushes should be soaked for up to an hour in a lice-killing solution to destroy any bugs or eggs still attached. Others suggest that washing them thoroughly in hot, soapy water is sufficient. There is no need to keep treated children away from school, as the dead lice and eggs are not infectious. All the treatments are available on prescription.

Body lice infestation needs to be treated with lotions that kill the lice, and all clothing and bedding need to be disinfected by machine washing using the hot cycle. Adult body lice like to sit in the seams of clothing, so it is sensible to iron the seams carefully after the machine wash. Alternatively, clothes can be dusted with a lice-killing powder. If it is at all realistic, the best solution is to throw the clothes away.

What should I expect?

Head lice do not cause any serious disease, but itching is a common symptom. Bites from body lice are even more likely to cause itching. This can be relieved by antihistamines and steroid creams. Scratching can damage the skin and can open the way to bacterial infection that can cause weeping and crusting of the scalp. If this happens it needs to be treated with antibiotics.

What else can I do?

If you want to check for head lice in your child's hair, use a fine-toothed comb and – unless your child has tight curly hair – plenty of conditioner. This makes it a lot easier to put the comb through. Tight curly hair is best combed without previous treatment with conditioner. It is a good idea to check this if there is a local head lice epidemic in your child's school. You will detect any infestation early and regular fine combing can itself get rid of the lice, but it is very labour-intensive. Don't leave any conditioner on the hair when you apply the lotion to kill the lice as the conditioner will actually keep the lotion away from the hair.

When treating the affected child follow the instructions on the packet and remember to treat the whole household, even if they have no symptoms, to reduce the chances of re-infestation. Even so, it is not unusual to get recurrent infestation and the whole process then needs to be repeated. You should check with a doctor before treating any children under two or using the shampoos and lotions on women who are trying to conceive, or are pregnant or breastfeeding.

Limping

What is it?

Small children are often falling over or bumping into things, and pain from some minor trauma during play is the usual cause of a limp. There are many other possible causes, however, some of which are very rare. These include:

- septic joints
- bone infection
- inadequate blood supply to a bone or part of a bone
- displacement of the growing part of the bone
- tumours
- juvenile arthritis
- congenital dislocation of the hip
- unequal leg length
- diseases of the nervous or muscular systems
- cerebral palsy
- psychological disturbance.

What action should I take?

Even though a minor injury will quickly recover with rest, a child with a new limp should be seen early by a doctor because of the danger of delayed diagnosis and treatment of the less common but potentially serious causes. If the limp is the result of a recent injury, take your child to the nearest accident and emergency department. Otherwise, visit your GP.

What should I expect?

It can be hard to diagnose the cause of a limp quickly. Young children may not be able to tell you or the doctor exactly where it hurts, and it may be difficult to decide whether the pain is located in muscle, bone, or joints. Your doctor will do a full examination, looking for tender spots and checking the range of movement at each joint. Depending on what this shows, your child will either be kept under review until the limp disappears, or will be sent for a number of investigations such as bone x-rays or scans.

If a joint, usually the knee, is swollen with fluid, a fine needle will be inserted into the affected area and some of the fluid will be sucked up into a syringe and checked in the laboratory for signs of infection or for types of arthritis (see page 149). Children with bacterial joint infections are usually very ill and feverish. Children whose limp has a psychological cause walk bizarrely and the clinical findings tend to change each time they are examined. If the limp persists your child is likely to be referred for specialist orthopaedic advice.

Measles

What is it?

Measles is a viral infection found throughout the world. Its main features are chest disease and a rash. In the UK there used to be regular epidemics every two years and 90 per cent of children had had measles by the time they were ten years old, 50 per cent of them by the time they were four. The mass immunisation programme introduced in 1968 interrupted this cycle. Now over 90 per cent of children in the UK are immunised against measles and it has become a rare disease in the UK, but across the world between one and two million children still die from measles every year.

When a child with measles coughs, sneezes or speaks, invisible airborne droplets of moisture containing the measles virus are produced. A child with measles is very infectious from three to five days before the rash appears and for a further four days after. Susceptible children, who have neither been immunised nor yet had measles, will almost always develop the disease after inhaling these infected droplets.

Immunity after infection is lifelong.

What action should I take?

Although protective proteins (antibodies) are passed from mother to baby across the placenta, these will protect your baby against measles only for the first 6-12 months of life. If you haven't had measles but you have had the jab, the antibodies produced after immunisation will protect your baby in the same way but probably for a shorter time.

It is therefore important to have your child immunised against measles (page 50).

What should I expect?

Measles has an average incubation period (the time between infection by the virus and the appearance of the illness) of 10-14 days, although it may be as short as 7 days or as long as 18 days. Illness starts with a sudden high fever, persistent croupy cough, runny nose, catarrhal chestiness and sore, runny eyes. Inside the mouth the tonsils are red and swollen and may have some white patches on them. The gums may also be coated with a thin grey film. The roof of the mouth and the insides of the cheeks are a discoloured, dirty, blotchy dark red. Tiny white pinpoint specks, like grains of sand on a velvet background, may be seen on the inside of the cheeks, just opposite the molar teeth, before the characteristic skin rash appears. These are called Koplik's spots and are found only in measles. Your child will be miserable and irritable. Diarrhoea is common, especially in young children. The high fever may provoke febrile fits (page 31). The symptoms tend to be worse in very young children and teenagers.

The rash appears after three to four days of the illness. It starts behind the ears and around the hairline, and spreads over the face and down the body during the next three days. The dusky red rash may become blotchy and swollen on the face. Over the body the individual red spots may run together to form large blotches. With the appearance of the rash all the symptoms become worse and the child becomes much more miserable. The temperature also rises, quite commonly to about 40°C (104°F). About four days after the rash first appears it will begin to fade in the same order in which it first spread, from the face downwards, and the worst of the illness is over within ten days or so. Sometimes a small number of blood cells may leak out of tiny blood vessels in the skin and give the rash a brown staining. This discoloration will persist for a week or two. If there are no complications the child will be getting back to normal within two weeks.

However, the measles virus attacks numerous body sites and the following complications can occur:

- ear infection in about 20 per cent of under-fives and 5 per cent of older children – the signs of this are increased misery, persistent fever and pulling at the ear
- diarrhoea in about 15 per cent of under-fives and 3 per cent of older children
- pneumonia in about 10 per cent of under-fives and 3 per cent of older children – the signs of this are persistent fever and cough
- inflammation of the brain (encephalitis) in the second week of the illness in about one in every 1000 cases – the signs of this are continued fever, drowsiness and disorientation.

Up to half of the children who develop measles encephalitis die, and up to half of the survivors have persistent neurological problems such as deafness and mental retardation.

Some time after they have been ill with measles, one in 250,000 children will show signs of a persistent measles infection of the nervous system, probably because of some abnormal immune response, or lack of response, to the measles virus. On average this happens eight years after the acute illness, but it can happen at any time between a few months to 20 years afterwards. It usually happens in children who had their attack of measles in the first two years of life. It starts slowly but is relentless and untreatable. The child or young adult shows intellectual deterioration and personality changes, develops clumsy movements and convulsions, and dies after several months to two years of a harrowing illness.

Some children are not immunised because they are at increased risk of severe measles – for example, those who have been receiving treatment for cancers. If they are exposed to someone with measles, they should be given the measles vaccine within 72 hours or, where appropriate, a special anti-measles antibody preparation in the form of a drip.

There is no specific anti-viral drug for measles so any treatment is directed at the symptoms – such as paracetamol for fever – and at any complication – such as antibiotics for a secondary bacterial pneumonia or ear infection. Nor is there any specific treatment for measles encephalitis although the hospital will provide pain relief and general care.

What else can I do?

Since children are highly infectious before the measles rash appears there is little to be gained from strict isolation procedures. You should, however, keep your child away from school until at least four to five days after the rash comes out. In any case, the child is unlikely to be well enough to go to school for at least two weeks.

Well-nourished children in developed countries need nursing rather than drugs as treatment for measles. Keep them in bed during the first few days of fever and keep giving drinks – any that they prefer. During the fever, tepid sponging may make them feel more comfortable. If after this stage they want to get up they should be allowed to do so.

WHAT TO DO IN AN EMERGENCY

Measles can be a severe illness and one in every 70 children who develops it will be admitted to hospital. You need take no emergency action yourself, but be aware of the possible complications and consult your doctor early if you suspect measles.

Meningitis

What is it?

Meningitis is an infection of the meninges, the membranes that cover the surface of the brain. There are a whole host of viruses and bacteria which can cause meningitis. **Viral meningitis** is often mild and many sufferers and their parents have no idea that they have a form of meningitis; or it can be like 'flu – a full recovery can be expected. It can, however, also cause a blinding headache and make the child extremely miserable. Sometimes it can be very difficult for the doctor to differentiate between viral and bacterial meningitis and usually the child needs to be admitted to hospital.

Most **bacterial meningitis** is caused by one of two infections: pneumococcal or meningococcal. (*Haemophilus influenzae* meningitis has virtually become a disease of the past thanks to immunisation – see page 49.) The meningococcal bug is often responsible for local outbreaks and attracts large amounts of worrying publicity, though isolated cases are more common. It is rather odd in that it can live at the back of the nose of otherwise apparently healthy people for a long period of time. For reasons that are not entirely clear it can become virulent, enter the bloodstream (causing blood poisoning or septicaemia) and invade many sites of the body, including the meninges, causing meningitis. The meningococcus is more likely to cause serious illness in a child under one year of age. Severe meningococcal disease may also be the first sign that children have something wrong with their immune system, impairing their ability to fight infection.

The septicaemic type of infection with the meningococcal bacteria is a potentially devastating illness and sometimes the affected child is gravely ill. Like the diphtheria bug, meningococcal bacteria release a powerful toxin which does the damage. In some forms of meningococcal infection a child can be well one moment and critically ill within a few hours. It is this which makes the meningococcal infection one of the most feared forms of infection and one which needs immediate identification and treatment.

If you suspect meningitis do not be afraid or embarrassed to create a fuss. Early recognition both by parents and doctors saves lives in this potentially fatal condition.

What should I expect?
Viral meningitis usually has quite an abrupt onset. Your child may go to school as normal but be sent home later in the day suffering from headache and vomiting. Sometimes the attack may start with a short 'flu-like illness, followed by one to two days of feeling vaguely unwell, before the headache begins. Neck pain and fever, between 99° and 101° (37.2° and 38.3°), are almost always

WHAT TO DO IN AN EMERGENCY

The main symptoms of meningococcal meningitis are:

- severe headache and generally feeling ill
- fever
- vomiting
- intolerance of bright light
- drowsiness.

Children with the meningococal bug usually become ill over one to two days, but symptoms can increase slowly over one to two weeks, or suddenly over hours. Your child may develop a **rapidly spreading pin prick or purpuric rash** – this is like a bruising of the skin and won't fade if you run your fingers over it or press on it with a glass. He or she may also suddenly become **unresponsive** after complaining of headache and fever.

In either case, call your doctor who may immediately start antibiotic treatment before getting your child admitted to hospital. If you can't reach your doctor, take your child to the nearest hospital accident and emergency department **urgently**.

present. The temperature stays up for three to five days, but rarely lasts longer than a week. Vomiting is common and often children complain of a vague tummy ache. Most recover within two weeks.

There is no specific treatment for viral meningitis. Usually pain relief (paracetamol) for the headache is all that is needed. Children will recover fully after a few days.

Bacterial meningitis has all the features of the viral form but is more severe. To start with your child may be just generally unwell with a headache, neck stiffness and general body ache. After 12 hours or so it becomes clear that this is something more serious, with high temperature, vomiting and a very severe headache. Occasionally, the meningitis may progress very rapidly and within a few hours the child is critically ill.

The exception to this characteristic pattern of events is bacterial meningitis in infancy. For the first three days the only sign may be that your baby is just not well. A baby cannot complain of headache, but may not feed well, may be listless or irritable, and may dislike being handled. A few days can pass before you realise that your baby is not just a bit off-colour but is really quite ill. The soft spot at the front of the head – the fontanelle – may bulge, but this certainly is not seen in every case. A cry that the parents recognise as unusual is probably a more reliable sign of something serious. The only unequivocal way to diagnose meningitis is by a lumbar puncture, which is an examination of the cerebrospinal fluid which circulates around the brain and spinal cord. A sample of this fluid is obtained by inserting a fine needle into the lower back and allowing a small volume to drain off. The fluid sample is sent to the laboratory where the particular bug can be identified. If bacterial meningitis is suspected, treatment will be started before the lab results become available and will be altered if necessary when the results arrive.

Treatment will involve an antibiotic drip starting as soon as possible and continuing for seven to ten days. Two to three days can go by before there are clear signs of recovery. Severely ill children, especially those with meningitis and septicaemia, may need to be treated in an intensive care unit.

Although the majority of survivors from bacterial meningitis make a complete recovery, there is a risk of permanent complications such as deafness, spasticity, learning difficulties and behavioural problems. Of these, deafness is the most common and after they have recovered all children are referred for hearing tests.

Close contacts of children with **meningococcal meningitis** are at increased risk of getting the illness themselves. The meningococcal bug is spread by small airborne droplets from the back of the nose of someone with meningitis or from someone who just has the bacteria living there harmlessly. If disease is going to occur, it will emerge within two to ten days after contact. Studies show that in 1 per cent of families who have a child with meningococcal meningitis, a second case will occur in the same household in the next month. All close contacts will be given appropriate antibiotics to reduce this risk. The aim is to get rid of the bug at the back of the nose.

There is no vaccine that protects against all the different types of meningococcal bacteria. Immunisation against meningococcal types A and C is available but protection lasts only a few years, and the group C part is effective only among children over two years old. There is no vaccine against type B – which causes most cases of meningococcal meningitis in the UK. Vaccination will be recommended for people other than close contacts only if there is a local outbreak of meningococcal meningitis caused by types A or C. Immediate family contacts will be given treatment by the hospital staff caring for the child. Others will be advised and treated by public health doctors and nurses or their family doctors.

What else can I do?

Haemophilus influenzae infection can be prevented by the Hib vaccination given in the first year of life. Make sure that your child is fully immunised (see Chapter 3). Since the introduction of the Hib vaccine the incidence of *Haemophilus influenzae* type B (Hib) meningitis has plunged dramatically.

It is important to bear the possibility of meningitis in mind when your child is ill, but also to keep the fear of meningitis in perspective: a GP will probably see only one case of meningitis every five years. On the other hand there are between about 1,200 and 2,000 cases of meningococcal meningitis every year in the UK and most of these are young children.

Mumps

What is it?

Mumps is a viral infection which is easily passed on by airborne droplets or by direct contact with saliva. Anyone with mumps is most infectious about two days before feeling unwell, but the virus can be found in saliva from six days before to nine days after the appearance of the characteristic swelling of the glands around the jaw. The incubation period (the time from getting the infection to the appearance of the symptoms) averages about 18 days with a range of two to three weeks.

Mumps is rare in children under two years old and is most common in those between five and nine. Before 1988, when the mumps vaccine became part of the routine childhood immunisation programme, there were regular epidemics in the UK about every three years, with the highest infection rates occurring in winter and spring.

What action should I take?

As many as three or four out of every ten mumps infections are very mild and produce no signs of illness. But these symptom-less

223

people are still infectious, so the only way for you to protect your children against mumps is to have them immunised at about 12 to 15 months and again at four years with the combined MMR vaccine (see Chapter 3). There is no specific treatment for mumps.

What should I expect?

Mumps is usually a mild illness but a few children will have significant pain, generally feel rotten and may suffer various complications (see below). It usually starts in a non-specific way, with any combination of fever, headache, sore throat or abdominal pain, for one to two days.

About seven out of ten children with mumps have infection and inflammation in one of the parotid glands. These saliva-producing glands sit on the cheeks, just in front of the ears and over the angle of the jaws. Initially, children may complain of earache, tenderness over the parotid gland and pain on chewing.

A couple of days later one or both parotid glands swell rapidly and painfully. Where only one gland seems to be involved, the other commonly follows suit within five days. The skin over the gland may be flushed and feel warm. With moderate to severe inflammation of the gland, children may be reluctant to open their mouths because of the pain and swelling. Blockage of the outflow tube from the gland to the mouth prevents the normal flow of saliva, resulting in a dry mouth. Other salivary glands lying just under the jawbone also start getting swollen and painful in about one in ten children. This glandular swelling increases over three days and then disappears over the next week.

Before the introduction of mass immunisation for mumps, 1,500 children were admitted to hospital each year with complications. Most of these admissions were for mumps meningitis (inflammation of the tissues covering the brain) or mumps encephalitis (inflammation of the brain itself). Such cases are mostly very mild and usually occur a few days after the parotid swelling. A more severe and permanent complication is deafness, although this is still rare. Children may also suffer arthritis and painful inflammation of the breast tissue.

Other complications tend to occur mainly in older children – for example, the testicles can become inflamed and fertility can be reduced, but this is extremely rare before puberty. It has, however, been reported in prepubescent boys, who usually have testicular pain, swelling and tenderness about four to five days after the salivary gland swells. Although symptoms may be mild, it is more usual to have very painful testicles and a worsening of the general illness with high fever, chills and muscle aches. Usually just one testicle is affected but the second one can follow the same pattern a day or two later. Symptoms settle after about four days.

What else can I do?
Bed rest and simple pain relief such as paracetamol are the mainstays of treatment. In terms of diet, children may prefer food that can be chewed easily. The most effective action you can take is to make sure that your child is immunised.

Nose bleed

What is it?
A nose bleed is a swelling and bursting of the tiny blood vessels in the lining of the nose. The medical term for a nose bleed is epistaxis. Nose bleeds are common in children and rarely serious, but they may keep on happening. The lining of the central part of the nose – the septum – has small blood vessels near the surface whose job is to act like a radiator, moistening and warming the air before it reaches the lungs. But sometimes they can swell and burst, usually caused by a mild infection, nose-picking or an allergy such as hay fever. Very rarely nose bleeds can be the result of a blood-clotting disorder such as haemophilia.

What action should I take?
Gently pinch the soft lower part of the nose between your thumb and index finger for ten minutes, without letting go. Then gently release. Do not blow the nose or poke tissues inside.

What should I expect?
A nose bleed should stop if you follow the procedure outlined above, but you can expect further bleeds over the next few days until the lining of the nose has fully healed. If the nose bleed is prolonged or severe, take your child to see a doctor. The nose may have to be packed with gauze for 24 hours. Afterwards your child

will probably be invited to see an ear, nose and throat specialist who may recommend cautery-burning – using heat to destroy the tissues in the area responsible for bleeding. This can be done with a chemical applied with a cotton bud, or with an electrical cautery. The chemical method is simpler but may have only temporary effects. The electrical method is for more severe problems but means that your child would need a short general anaesthetic.

What else can I do?
Don't worry: nose bleeds in children are not usually serious and will probably stop happening as the child grows. Make sure that any allergies are treated, and consider pet allergies and hay fever as possible underlying causes.

Penile and foreskin problems

It is often mothers who are left to sort out problems with their little boys' genitals and personal hygiene, and fathers may have forgotten what to expect. Many parents are embarrassed at seeking medical advice over what they think is a trivial matter. However, do not be shy about asking the health visitor or your GP about problems to do with your son's penis or foreskin. See also the section on 'Testicular problems' on page 239.

1: Phimosis and paraphimosis

What are they?
A **phimosis** is an abnormally small hole at the end of the foreskin, the hood of skin which covers the head of the penis (the glans). At birth the foreskin is usually unretractable but by the age of four the vast majority of boys can retract their foreskin. Some boys are born with an unusually tight foreskin, or pieces of tissue might connect it to the head of the penis, making it difficult to retract. If there is a phimosis there will be a poor urinary stream and the foreskin will swell like a balloon as it acts as a reservoir when urine is being passed. Phimosis can be caused by using excessive force as you try to retract the foreskin and by infections around this area.

A **paraphimosis** is when the retracted foreskin is trapped in the retracted position, causing painful swelling of the head of the penis. It may have to be relieved as an emergency.

Infections around the foreskin are relatively common, resulting in redness and swelling and possibly a discharge of pus.

What action should I take?

Do not attempt to retract the foreskin forcibly as you may damage the tissues, resulting in a phimosis. If you suspect a paraphimosis, seek urgent medical help either from your GP or go to your nearest accident and emergency department. Infections around the foreskin area can be prevented by keeping the area clean. If an infection does not settle after a few days, seek medical advice.

What should I expect?

If a phimosis is a problem, circumcision may be recommended – see below. If a paraphimosis cannot be reduced and the foreskin not replaced, it may have to be done under an anaesthetic. This involves reducing either by simple pressure or by making a slit in the foreskin. This is often followed up by a circumcision at a later date.

2: Hypospadias

What is it?

Hypospadias is a condition in which the urinary opening is not at the tip of the penis, but develops on the underside of the shaft. This can affect about one in 350 male babies and so is relatively common. In a similar but rarer condition called epispadias, the opening is on the topside of the shaft of the penis.

What action should I take?

Hypospadias should be diagnosed at birth, if not by the parents then by the doctor doing the routine baby checks. It is always worth a look to make sure that the 'hole' occurs at the right point.

What should I expect?

There are varying degrees of hypospadias. Many men have a very small deviation away from the tip which causes them no inconvenience and is frequently discovered only accidentally at a routine medical examination in adulthood. However, in some children the degree of hypospadias is quite severe and in these cases an operation can be done to correct the problem. The timing of the surgery very much depends on the severity and distress caused by the condition.

What else can I do?
Do not arrange for your baby to have a circumcision before a surgical procedure to correct the hypospadias. The foreskin may be required as part of the surgical reconstruction.

3: Circumcision

What is it?
Circumcision is the removal of the foreskin. This may be required for religious reasons but there are very few medical reasons for having a circumcision. Occasionally, however, it may be needed in cases of phimosis (see above) and your doctor may suggest a circumcision if there is a paraphimosis. It is true that circumcised boys rarely go on to develop a cancer of the penis, but this type of cancer is in any case quite rare.

What action should I take?
If your son is having a circumcision for religious reasons, it is possible that a non-medical person may perform it. You must check that this person is experienced in such procedures, although you may find that he successfully performs more circumcisions that do most doctors! You should also check that all equipment is sterilised.

What should I expect?
Most foreskin problems do not require a circumcision, so if your doctor suggests that your son should have one, make sure you understand why he or she considers it necessary. Circumcision is a reasonably safe procedure, usually carried out under a general anaesthetic, but it carries a risk of subsequent infection and bleeding from the wound.

What else can I do?
If your son does have a circumcision, make sure you get clear instructions about how to dress the wound afterwards.

MASTURBATION

All children – girls as well as boys – masturbate from a very early age and erections are common even in small boys. There is no harm in masturbation. The only problems arise from a feeling of guilt associated with masturbation, usually because children do not understand why they feel the pleasant sensations that the action brings. If you find your child masturbating, it is important you do not reinforce his or her guilt.

Pneumonia

See **chickenpox**, page 160; **respiratory tract infection** (below); **whooping cough**, page 248.

Rash

See **allergy**, page 146; **chickenpox**, page 160; **eczema**, page 184; **impetigo**, page 210; **measles**, page 216; **meningitis**, page 219; **ringworm**, page 233; **scabies**, page 234; **slapped cheek syndrome**, page 238.

Red eye

See **conjunctivitis**, page 165; **measles**, page 216.

Respiratory tract infection

What is it?

A multitude of names is used to describe what happens when an infection descends from the upper airways such as the windpipe to the deeper parts of the lungs within the chest cavity. There is considerable overlap between the conditions and the symptoms are often the same although there may be a difference in the severity of the illness. This depends on the nature of the underlying condition, the general health of the child and the virulence of the underlying cause. There are a whole host of organisms which can cause a chest infection and part of the treatment involves working out which bug is responsible.

Colds
See page 27.

Bronchitis
The bronchi branch off from the windpipe and are the main tubes or airways that transport air to and from the lungs. They are constructed from several layers of tissue but it is the inner layers that are affected most. In an episode of acute bronchitis it is often an infection from higher up the respiratory tract – perhaps a cold or a 'flu-like virus – which descends down the respiratory tree. In its wake it causes inflammation of the lining of the tubes and encourages the glands lining the inner surface of the bronchi to secrete excess mucus.

Initially the child may have a mild cold which, after a couple of days, may progress to a cough, sometimes with lots of catarrh and phlegm. This phlegm may be discoloured (often greeny yellow), indicating a bacterial infection. Sometimes there is a temperature and occasionally there can be wheezing. Bronchitis should not be confused with bronchiolitis (page 28).

Wheezing is associated with asthma (page 151) but it is not unique to asthma and can occur with bronchitis. Wheezing is caused by an obstruction in the flow of air through the respiratory tubes, particularly the smaller tubes in the lungs. The obstruction occurs as the tubes go into spasm and get congested with swollen linings and excess secretions. Babies are more likely than adults to wheeze because their airway tubes are proportionately smaller than those of adults. It is not uncommon for someone to have recurrent episodes of wheezing as a child and eventually grow out of the problem. Many wheezing episodes are associated with infection, but it is important to be aware that for some children with repeated episodes of wheezing asthma may be the underlying cause.

Bronchitis is often caused by a virus infection, so many children with a short, sharp attack of bronchitis will get better by themselves as the body starts to fight the infection with its own natural defences. If the bronchitis is caused by a bacterial infection, your child may need treatment.

Pneumonia
Pneumonia is an inflammation of the lung tissue itself. It can be caused by bacteria, viruses or, rarely, a fungal infection. Again, it is

commonly associated with an upper respiratory tract infection which descends deeper into the lungs. Although any child could have pneumonia, it is more common in children whose immunity is lowered, for example those receiving chemotherapy for cancer (page 155) or those with an underlying chest abnormality such as cystic fibrosis (page 170).

The symptoms are often similar to those of acute bronchitis although children with pneumonia may be more ill and have some difficulty breathing. Young children and babies may just seem unwell and have no obvious chest symptoms. The doctor might not be able to diagnose pneumonia from a physical examination but it will show up on a chest x-ray, so this is a really essential test when the doctor cannot find any obvious cause for a child's illness.

Tuberculosis
In the recent past tuberculosis was on the decline and considered a rarity. That is no longer the case, although it still is not common. Tuberculosis can affect otherwise well children and you should be particularly suspicious if your child is unwell following contact with someone known to have tuberculosis. The symptoms can include cough, fever, loss of appetite and weight loss. For more information on immunisation against tuberculosis see Chapter 3.

Bronchiectasis
This is much less common now than it used to be but may still occur. Bronchiectasis is associated with damage to the bronchi and leads to enlargement of these tubes. It can follow a nasty pneumonia. The symptoms are coughing, producing a lot of sputum and failure to thrive.

What action should I take?
You know your child best and you can tell how unwell he or she is. If a child has a runny nose with a mild cough and is not that unwell, it would not be unreasonable to try to manage this yourself. Cough medicines may be soothing but otherwise have little if any practical value. Most are not available on prescription. The simplest and cheapest form of treatment involves warm drinks and paracetamol to relieve a fever.

If you are unsure whether to see a doctor or not, then go for reassurance, but if your child is otherwise well, there is no reason why you shouldn't just wait and watch what happens; most children will get better by themselves. If there is no improvement after two or three days, or if there is a significant deterioration, get medical advice.

What should I expect?
The doctor will ask questions about the history of the illness, examine the chest and listen with a stethoscope to hear the quality of the breath sounds, and make a general assessment of the child's overall current health.

Occasionally, and especially if the child is ill, a chest x-ray will be requested. This will show the state of the heart and lungs and is particularly good at picking up pneumonia. It will not normally show any signs of bronchitis. If a child is admitted to hospital the staff will try to work out which particular bug is causing the problem. This may involve blood tests and culturing sputum.

Antibiotics are of no use in treating viral infections, but in practice it is not always easy to differentiate between viral and bacterial infections. The more ill the child, the more likely he or she is to be given antibiotics.

What else can I do?
Both during and after the illness you can make sure your child has enough to drink and that his or her temperature is kept under control. Children and babies can survive quite happily without food

---

WHAT TO DO IN AN EMERGENCY

Chest infections rarely cause a sudden and dramatic deterioration but it can happen sometimes. Signs to look out for are:

- a high temperature
- obvious difficulty in breathing
- drowsiness and even confusion.

If this happens you need to get medical help urgently: either speak to your GP and arrange an urgent consultation at home or in the surgery, or take your child to the nearest accident and emergency department.

---

for some time, but fluids are indispensable. If your child won't or can't drink and is becoming dehydrated as a result of the chest infection, then that alone is a reason for hospital admission. Contrary to popular belief, taking a child outside does not bring on a chest infection or delay recovery. A breath of fresh air and a trip outside the house can be a real morale booster to both child and carer.

Ringworm

What is it?
Ringworm is a fungal infection found throughout the world and defined by the body part affected, such as the scalp, body, groin, hand, foot or nail – so, for example, you might hear of scalp ringworm or nail ringworm. The infection is spread by direct contact with someone who has the infection or by contact with that person's skin scales. This could happen as a result of sharing combs, hairbrushes or hats (scalp ringworm) or from contact with a changing-room floor (foot ringworm).

What action should I take?
Mild body and groin ringworm will respond to anti-fungal creams or ointments. More severe or chronic skin problems, scalp and nail ringworm may need to be treated with anti-fungal tablets or medicines. You may have to give your child the tablets for some weeks or even months.

Reinfection should be prevented by looking for and treating the source of the infection, which is usually another child, adult or family pet. Everyone should have their own combs and hairbrush to avoid sharing.

What should I expect?
People with ringworm have an expanding rash with a scaly edge. Scalp infection occurs mostly in children, usually as one or more oval patches, although it can progress to the whole scalp. Hairs are damaged and break off near the skin surface. Rarely the hair follicles become filled with pus and the ensuing scarring can cause permanent hair loss.

Body ringworm is usually an obvious red scaling area that heals in the centre as its edges expand. Groin infection is found in the groin skin folds and creases, often spreading down the thighs. Ringworm on the hands or feet tends to be very scaly, with cracking of the skin. The spaces between the toes are often particularly badly affected. Infected nails become opaque, discoloured and brittle, and the entire nail may flake away.

What else can I do?

Do everything you can to prevent reinfection (see above).

Scabies

What is it?

Scabies is caused by the scabetic mite burrowing into the upper layer of the skin. The female lays her eggs in the burrow. These hatch into larvae (baby mites), move to the surface, mature in about three weeks, mate and repeat the cycle. Infection is spread from person to person through direct skin contact. The mites are attracted by the warmth generated by skin contact and burrow into the skin of the new host. They are transmitted easily by holding hands or sharing a bed. Contrary to popular belief they are not spread by clothing or bedding.

What action should I take?

Your doctor will prescribe creams or lotions that will kill the mites. The whole skin surface except the head and face must be treated. You need to make especially sure that you get enough lotion on your child's hands and feet, being careful to reapply it after handwashing. The cream or lotion can be washed off after 12-24 hours. Occasionally, a second treatment is needed two to three days later. Everyone in the household must be treated.

Bedding and clothing do not need any special washing, but should be washed in hot water at the end of therapy. They do not harbour any mites.

What should I expect?

The infection itself causes no symptoms. The intense itching results from a sensitivity to the mites or the eggs, so it starts only about two to three weeks after the initial infection. Similarly, it can take three weeks for the sensitivity to abate and therefore the itching to disappear after appropriate treatment has killed the mites. Itching is worse at night.

The scabetic rash is a combination of the burrow (a pinhead-sized blister with a short accompanying line), small raised lumps, scratch marks and an eczema-like reaction. It is usually found on the fingers, especially in the web spaces, around the armpits, wrists, elbows, waist, buttocks, genitalia, groin and ankles. In a young child the rash is often seen on the palms, soles, head and neck, but you still need to apply the lotion only from the neck down because the scabies mite is not found above the neck – the rash is a secondary phenomenon. With older children the head and back are usually spared. If a bacterial infection settles into the affected skin, your doctor can prescribe appropriate antibiotics.

What else can I do?
Calamine lotion can be used to relieve itching.

Scaly skin

See **ringworm**, page 233.

Scoliosis

What is it?
Normally the spine is straight, when looked at from behind, but in scoliosis there is a curve to one side. In most cases the cause is unknown but scoliosis does tend to run in families. About 5 per cent of scoliosis is known to occur in association with other conditions such as bony spinal abnormalities, a short leg, muscular dystrophies and rare inherited diseases of the nervous system.

What action should I take?
Because of the genetic risk, if scoliosis occurs in one child, all the other children in the family should be examined by a doctor and then x-rayed if there is any concern that scoliosis may be present.

What should I expect?
A slight curve of the spine is not unusual in infancy. This is postural – in other words, it is dependent on the position the baby adopts – and disappears when the baby is held suspended. There is

no bony deformity, and by the age of one or two it will have gone completely.

A **postural scoliosis** in the older child shows as a mild curve that straightens with forward bending. This will correct itself and needs no treatment.

Scoliosis is more common in girls during adolescence, which is a time of rapid growth. The scoliosis eventually corrects itself in most cases, but these children must be regularly reviewed. The scoliosis may progress and need an operation.

Structural scoliosis is more serious. Here, the bony vertebrae that make up the spine are rotated. The scoliosis tends to increase until the spine stops growing. Small curves usually need no treatment, but children can be given exercises to help keep the back supple, as well as supports and splints to help prevent the curves getting worse; surgery is necessary when the scoliosis is severe and progressive.

What else can I do?
Be aware of your children's posture as they are growing and if you have any concerns get them checked by a doctor.

Sickle-cell disease

What is it?
Sickle-cell disease is an inherited condition causing a specific type of anaemia. It is found in people of African racial origin. If both parents have passed on the faulty gene, the child will suffer from sickle-cell anaemia. The result is an abnormal haemoglobin which causes red blood cells to develop a crescent shape when they are low in oxygen (the so-called sickle). If the child has inherited only one abnormal gene, coupled with one normal copy from the other parent, he or she will have the sickle-cell trait. People with the sickle-cell trait usually have no symptoms but they are carriers and may pass the rogue gene to their children. The trait is found in about 7–9 per cent of African-Americans.

What action should I take?
See your doctor if your child is pale or you suspect anaemia or, especially, if there is a family history of the condition.

What should I expect?

Sickle-cell anaemia often appears during a baby's first year as pallor, listlessness and mild jaundice. The onset of symptoms is delayed until the abnormal adult blood has replaced the foetal blood of the infant, which normally takes place over the first few months. In some cases there are recurrent crises where the blood cells break down with acute symptoms such as severe abdominal pain and rigidity, pain in the loins, limb pains, localised paralyses and convulsions. Painful swellings of the fingers and feet may develop as the small bones are deprived of vital blood supplies when the sickle-cells stick together and block small blood vessels. X-rays will show severe bone destruction as a result. Chronic anaemia interferes with growth and nutrition so that the child is often stunted in later years. Enlargement of the spleen may be marked and gallstones may develop. Children with the condition are also at greater risk of catching serious infections.

There is no specific treatment or cure for sickle-cell disease. Instead, the symptoms are treated and blood transfusions are frequently required for anaemia. In a severe crisis, the child may have to go into hospital for pain relief. Lack of fluids can make an attack more possible, so it is important to correct any dehydration quickly. With careful supervision and the use of blood transfusion many children with sickle-cell anaemia reach adult life. Patients of African extraction should ideally be tested for sickle-cell anaemia before they are given a general anaesthetic. Pre-operative preparation may require another blood transfusion.

What else can I do?

Always get help from a doctor if a child with sickle-cell disease becomes unwell, and make sure that you and your family have a good understanding of the condition. Make sure that your child has plenty of drinks so there is never a risk of dehydration. Some children with the disorder are at higher risk of contracting a pneumococcal infection so it is worth asking whether he or she would benefit from a pneumococcal vaccination.

Slapped cheek syndrome

What is it?

Slapped cheek syndrome is a viral infection, so called because of the characteristic bright red flush that it provokes on the cheeks of infected children. It is known worldwide and is very infectious, being transmitted between children by airborne droplets in breath. Epidemics in communities are common: they usually occur in the winter or spring and last from three to six months. Children usually catch the infection between the ages of five and 14. School outbreaks are common, again usually in the late winter or spring. The incubation period (the time between infection and the appearance of any symptoms), is around 14 days, but can be anything from 7 to 22 days. Once infected, children have lifelong protection against any repeat attacks.

What action should I take?

No specific anti-viral treatment exists. You can treat the fever with paracetamol and if the rash is particularly itchy, salty baths and calamine lotion may help. Most often the source of the infection cannot be traced. There is no need to keep your child away from school as most of those who are susceptible to catching the infection will have been exposed to the virus by the time your child is diagnosed.

What should I expect?

Research has shown that about half of infected children have no outward sign of illness. A few may have two to three days of mild illness with fever before developing the classic rash. For the rest, the rash is the first sign of the infection. It starts with a bright red flush on the cheeks. The edges of this fiery redness can be slightly raised, like a small bump, and the skin around the lips usually looks exaggeratedly pale. The facial rash becomes even more marked when the child comes into a warm room from outside.

One to four days later, a rash develops on the body, legs and arms. This is often itchy and starts as small red spots which join together to cover quite large areas of skin. The redness first clears from the centre of these larger blotches, giving a lace-like picture. Over the next few weeks, and sometimes for even longer, this lacy rash can come and go. Its reappearance is often provoked by sunlight or a hot bath.

Other symptoms are unusual, although about one in five children will complain of a headache and a small number may have painful joints.

What else can I do?

The virus attacks rapidly dividing cells, in particular the developing red blood cells in the bone marrow. This is not a problem for most healthy children, but it can cause a severe anaemia in children with certain inherited blood disorders like sickle-cell disease or thalassaemia. These children may need a blood transfusion. If your child has one of these blood disorders and develops any rash or feverish illness, followed by lethargy and pallor, contact your doctor immediately.

Sticky eye

See **conjunctivitis**, page 165.

Swollen glands

See **glandular fever**, page 205; **mumps**, page 223.

Swollen itchy eyes

See **conjunctivitis**, page 165; **hay fever**, page 201.

Swollen joints

See **arthritis**, page 149; **cancer**, page 155; **sickle-cell disease**, page 236.

Testicular problems

The most common problem involving the testicles is when one or both of a baby boy's testicles appears to be missing at birth. See pages 37-9 for more about undescended and retractile testicles. See also 'Penile and foreskin problems' on page 226.

1: Torsion of the testicle

What is it?

Torsion of the testicle describes a situation where the testicle twists on itself and in effect blocks off its own blood supply. Every case of testicular pain in boys and young men should be considered as torsion until proved otherwise. If the problem is not dealt with as a matter of urgency, the testicle will strangle itself, thus making the boy infertile.

What action should I take?
Any boy with a painful or swollen testicle should be seen urgently by a doctor. If you cannot get to your GP immediately, take your son to the nearest accident and emergency department.

What should I expect?
The pain is severe, local and sudden. Sometimes there is nausea and vomiting. There is also tenderness of the testicle and, later, scrotal swelling. Your son will need to go to hospital where a surgeon will probably explore the scrotum to unwind the testicle. The chances of a full recovery are high if the problem is caught early enough.

What else can I do?
The important thing is to act quickly: torsion of the testicles is a medical emergency.

2: Cancer of the testicles

This type of cancer is very rare in boys, although it can occur. If you or your son discover any new lumps or swellings in the testicles they should be examined by your GP.

Thalassaemia

What is it?
Thalassaemia is an inherited form of anaemia which is most common in people of Mediterranean, Asian and African origin. The thalassaemias are a mixed group of disorders affecting the manufacture of haemoglobin – the pigment in red blood cells which carries oxygen to the tissues of the body.

   If a child inherits the faulty gene from both parents the result is a severe anaemia. Those children who have inherited the gene from only one parent suffer only mild anaemia. The symptoms of thalassaemia cannot be detected in newborn babies because the chronic anaemia emerges only later in infancy. Paleness is a constant feature, the spleen increases in size throughout childhood and the liver may also enlarge.

Even with the best available treatment, it becomes obvious before puberty that the child has not grown normally. Boys in particular fail to mature at puberty. They may be short in stature and generally fail to thrive.

What action should I take?

If there is a family history of thalassaemia, you may benefit from genetic screening (see page 13). If your child is obviously pale, ask your doctor if he or she can arrange a blood test. If thalassaemia is diagnosed, find out which type it is: thalassaemia minor – where sufferers have only one copy of the faulty gene – does not require any treatment.

What should I expect?

The condition is diagnosed by blood tests and treated, if necessary, by regular blood transfusions. Unfortunately, regular blood transfusions mean that the body receives too much iron. This in turn can damage vital organs such as the heart. However, this can be overcome by taking a different drug at the same time to help get rid of excess iron. This delays or even prevents some of the more serious complications of iron overload.

What else can I do?

Any relatives, and especially the parents of an affected child, should have genetic counselling to assess their risk of developing or perpetuating the condition. If a couple planning to have a child are found to be at risk of carrying the faulty gene they need to have expert genetic counselling.

Tiredness

See **diabetes**, page 175; **glandular fever**, page 205; **sickle-cell disease**, page 236; **thalassaemia**, page 240.

Toddler's diarrhoea

What is it?

Toddlers aged from six months to two years can develop persistent diarrhoea, but remain well and happy and gain weight normally.

For some unknown reason, food travels through the stomach and bowels too quickly, causing undigested pieces of food such as peas, carrots and corn to be visible and identifiable in the diarrhoea.

What action should I take?

If your child has diarrhoea which doesn't settle it is usually worth visiting the doctor, even if the child seems well. Your doctor can check that there are no treatable or more serious causes of diarrhoea such as infections, parasites, colitis or food intolerances.

What can I expect?

As long as your child is healthy and is not suffering from tummy aches, then, after doing a physical examination, the doctor may simply reassure you that it is not a serious condition and will eventually settle down, but perhaps not until the child reaches the age of four or five. A sample of faeces may be sent to the laboratory to look for any bugs which can cause chronic diarrhoea. In toddler's diarrhoea, no bugs or infections are found.

What else can I do?

Continue to give your child a normal varied diet. If the diarrhoea continues over a long period of time, it may be worth monitoring your child's weight, either yourself or at the child health clinic. If any new symptoms develop or if your child fails to gain weight normally, the doctor may need to review the situation.

Tonsillitis and sore throats

What are they?

Tonsillitis literally means inflammation of the tonsils. These are tissues which are present at the back of the throat and are part of the body's normal defence mechanism, helping to prevent infections in the respiratory tract. Many people refer to any painful inflammatory condition of the back of the throat as tonsillitis, but there are other kinds of 'sore throat' including pharyngitis, an inflammation of the throat which causes symptoms similar to those of tonsillitis. Both these conditions can be caused by viruses and bacteria, although viruses are responsible for the majority of cases. Diphtheria is a rare but serious cause of sore throats, which are usually accompanied by swollen glands in the neck, a temperature and pain on swallowing – see page 178.

What action should I take?

Most sore throats are viral infections that require nothing more than treatment of the symptoms. Pain and fever are best dealt with by using a paracetamol or ibuprofen preparation specially designed for children. It is also important to keep feverish children cool with a fan and, if necessary, tepid sponging. If your child is ill or if the condition persists for more than 48 hours (24 hours in a younger child up to three or four), see your GP.

What should I expect?

If the tonsillitis is a true bacterial infection, your doctor will prescribe an antibiotic. The main treatment for simple, uncomplicated, bacterial tonsillitis is usually Phenoxymethyl penicillin (Penicillin V). There is no specific drug treatment for tonsillitis caused by a virus. Realistically, it is not feasible to tell just by looking at the throat which type of organism is causing the problem, so many doctors prescribe antibiotics on a 'best guess' policy without taking throat swabs to try to isolate the bug. It is only when the tonsils become so badly damaged by recurrent infections that they become the source of infection that it is necessary to remove them.

In some cases a tonsil may enlarge with infection to the extent that it can virtually block off the back of the throat, forming an abscess called a quinsy. If this happens your child will be quite ill and the situation has to be treated as an emergency. It may be necessary for the child to go to hospital for treatment with a high dose of an infusion of antibiotics or for an operation to deflate the abscess. The symptoms quickly get better after this but you may well be advised to have your child's tonsils removed at a later date, once all the inflammation has settled.

What else can I do?

A soothing cold drink such as milk may help some children with a sore throat, and using a straw may be more comfortable. Keep your child away from smoky environments as smoke is an obvious irritant.

Tummy ache

See **appendicitis**, page 148; **hepatitis and liver disease**, page 204; **mumps**, page 223.

Urinary tract infection

What is it?

The urinary tract is the system that filters the blood and excretes body waste products via the urine. It consists of the kidneys, the ureters, the bladder and the urethra. The kidneys actively filter the blood, maintain the water balance of the body and produce the urine. This is then passed to the pelvis of the kidney that acts as a funnel into the ureters. The ureters (one for each of the kidneys) are tubes connecting the kidneys to the bladder. The bladder stores the urine until it is ready to empty. The urine then passes through a tube called the urethra out of the body.

Any part of the urinary tract can get infected but the most common type of infection is in the bladder or urethra or both. Infections of the urinary tract are commonly caused by bacteria originating from the rectum. Occasionally, bacteria can enter the urinary system from the blood stream.

The anatomy of the urethra is probably the clue as to why girls get infected more frequently than boys: in girls the urethra is a very short tube that goes from the bladder to just inside the lips of the vagina, while boys have a longer urethra which opens further away from the body.

What action should I take?

See a doctor if you think your child may have a urinary tract infection. The symptoms in small children are fever, loss of appetite and generally looking ill – the symptoms of infection anywhere in the body, really. It is difficult to diagnose easily in small infants, and sometimes the diagnosis may be suggested by the fact that there are no signs in the other areas that commonly get infected, such as the respiratory tract. Older children often experience tummy pain, or pain or a burning sensation on passing urine (dysuria), or go to the toilet to pass urine more frequently than usual, or notice that the urine is discoloured.

What should I expect?

It is very important to diagnose and treat any infection adequately. Recurrent infections, particularly those which are not detected and treated, may lead to scarring of the kidney. In later life that can lead to high blood pressure or even kidney failure. In addition, the presence of an infection may be an indication that there is some kind of abnormality in the urinary system. A common and significant abnormality is urine reflux, whereby urine passes back up into the kidneys from the bladder. If there is infection in the urine, this can damage the kidneys.

Urinary tract infections are confirmed with laboratory testing of urine samples from the child. The urine is tested for the presence of bacteria, which are themselves tested for sensitivity to various antibiotics. The sample is obtained as a 'mid-stream urine' in older children – a clean collection of urine as the child is passing it – and as a 'supra-pubic stab' in small children, where a fine needle is passed into the bladder through the abdominal wall to collect the sample for testing. This is an essential method in very young infants, and is not traumatic or dangerous, although it is usually done at hospital. Any bacterial infection in the urine should be treated if possible with antibiotics.

If your child has a proven urinary tract infection it is likely that further tests may be done to look at the kidney and its associated apparatus to see whether there is an underlying abnormality.

What else can I do?

Encouraging your child to go to the toilet regularly and to drink plenty of fluids helps to flush out the urinary system and prevents bacteria taking root and multiplying. You may need to speak to the school authorities if your child has a problem with recurrent urinary tract infections and make sure there is easy access to toilet facilities. Teach your child to wipe his or her bottom from front to back. Doing it the other way will encourage bacteria to be pushed towards the genital area.

Urinary tract infection in adults may well respond to treatments other than antibiotics – for instance, several of the recommended herbal remedies appear to have a limited anti-bacterial action, and there is reasonable evidence to support a current vogue for using cranberry extracts to treat adult urinary tract infection. But it is not advisable to use complementary treatments for urinary tract infections in children: the risk of treating an infection in children inadequately is that they may go on to develop a more serious problem when they are older. On the other hand, there is no harm in using natural products such as cranberry juice as well as, but not instead of, antibiotics.

Verrucas and warts

What are they?

Warts are swellings of the outer layer of the skin and are caused by the human papilloma virus. They vary in size and may be uncomfortable, particularly if they occur on the feet, in which case they are known as plantar warts or verrucas. Warts also vary in shape and form, from small bumps on the skin to large cauliflower-like lumps often connected by a stalk to the skin. They are caused by a virus which is caught by direct contact with other people's warts or from wart residues left on towels or hard surfaces. They spread from site to site in the same child by direct contact or if the child scratches the wart surface and then touches another part of the body. Having said that, warts are not very infectious – it seems that some people are just more susceptible then others.

What action should I take?

Warts are not serious and do not always require treatment unless they are unsightly, uncomfortable or appear to be multiplying rapidly.

What should I expect?

In healthy children most warts will eventually disappear. If they don't there are several methods of dealing with them. Always get medical advice before treating any warts on the face, mouth or any other sensitive area as many of the treatments can cause local tissue damage and scarring.

Each method has its advantages and disadvantages. The regular application of a local medication, often containing salicylic acid, is the most common therapy. This destroys the horny skin layer and kills the virus. It is messy and involves regular applications of a toxic paint. The wart surface can then be 'sanded down' with a pumice stone to remove the destroyed layer. Eventually the wart disappears and the area under the wart starts to heal.

Another method is the use of liquid nitrogen or liquid carbon dioxide, applied as a spray on to the wart. This freezes the wart and a little bit of surrounding skin. The disadvantages of this method are that it may not work first time and may need several attempts over the course of a few months; it stings when the spray is applied (although even small children seem to tolerate this well); and it may cause a blister at the site which may then become infected. The advantages are that it is extremely effective and takes only a few seconds.

The other method in current use is surgical removal. This could mean cutting off the blood supply to the wart by tying it with surgical cotton, causing the wart to die and eventually fall off; or it could mean cutting out the wart under an anaesthetic. The cotton-tie method has the advantage of simplicity and speed, but is suitable only for those warts that have a stalk, and are not too small. Surgery is obviously a more traumatic option for children and is best avoided except as a last resort. If the wart recurs, it should probably be treated by freezing with liquid nitrogen, or surgical removal.

What else can I do?
Most warts die off naturally after a few years anyway, and some disappear spontaneously with no treatment, so just leaving them alone and avoiding the urge to do anything may be all that is required. Never try to treat a wart on the face without speaking to your doctor about it first.

Treat a verruca on the sole of the foot as indicated above; it may be reasonable to allow your child to resume swimming after a couple of weeks so long as the verruca is covered with a waterproof plaster.

Vomiting

See **gastro-enteritis**, page 195; **hepatitis and liver disease**, page 204; **meningitis**, page 219.

Weight loss

See **coeliac disease**, page 161; **diabetes**, page 175.

Wheezing and breathlessness

See **asthma**, page 151; **bronchitis**, page 230; **hay fever**, page 201; **pneumonia**, page 231.

Whooping cough

What is it?

Whooping cough, also known as pertussis, is a bacterial infection spread by airborne droplets. It is highly infectious when there is close contact between someone with the infection and a susceptible, unimmunised child. Children are most infectious in the first week of the illness, when the symptoms are indistinguishable from those of a bad cold, so you would not have known to isolate your child.

Whooping cough is found throughout the world, and epidemics occur every few years in countries without effective vaccination programmes. It is at its worst in the winter but never disappears entirely. Any age group can be attacked, but whooping cough is mainly a disease of infancy and childhood. Infection can be fatal, with most of the deaths being among babies and young children.

The spread of whooping cough in an institution where large numbers of children are living together may be minimised by giving antibiotics early on. There is, however, no evidence that antibiotic treatment protects any individual child in an ordinary family or school situation.

What action should I take?

You should consult your doctor if your child has any unusual or prolonged cough. Although whooping cough is the most likely cause of a cough that goes on and on, other important possibilities such as asthma need to be considered and either ruled out or confirmed using appropriate tests. Children with such a symptom may need a chest x-ray.

The coughing spasms of whooping cough often lead to vomiting, especially in babies. If this is a problem, try giving small amounts of food more frequently. If your child becomes blue around the lips or mouth during coughing, or appears to be choking, or you are frightened that he or she will stop breathing, you must see your doctor urgently.

What should I expect?

The incubation period (the time from infection to the appearance of symptoms) is about seven to ten days. The first catarrhal stage lasts about a week and at this point there is nothing to distinguish the infection from the ordinary coughs and colds of childhood. There may be a slight fever with an irritating, dry cough. However, rather than shaking off the cold, things get noticeably worse, the cough starts to come in bouts and the typical symptoms of whooping cough begin.

At this stage children suffer spasms of coughing which can last minutes. During these spasms their eyes will water and bulge, their faces turn red, or even blue, the veins on the head and neck swell, and saliva pours from their mouths. Not surprisingly, they look scared and many parents are frightened that their child will choke and stop breathing. At the end of a coughing bout a large intake of breath through a windpipe in spasm produces the typical 'whoop'. This may end the coughing bout or the child may go straight into another one without any relief.

In very young children and babies there may be no spasmodic coughing phase, just a prolonged catarrhal, cold-like illness. These children can still be very ill and even die. Older children may have only a mild spasmodic stage, often without the characteristic culminating whoop.

The spasms of severe coughing can last from one to four weeks, although there is usually some easing up after a fortnight. Bouts of coughing can carry on for about three months – whooping cough is sometimes called the 'hundred days cough'.

Although babies less than six months old are particularly at risk of dying from episodes of prolonged lack of breathing and a failure to breathe at the end of a coughing spasm, there are many other potential and serious complications, including brain damage from a lack of oxygen, bleeding into the eye, hernias, inhalation of vomit and pneumonia from a superimposed infection.

There is no cure for established whooping cough. The illness must run its natural course. Children who develop whooping cough may be given liquid feeds through a thin tube that passes through the nose and past the back of the throat to the stomach, or they may be given fluids through a drip, oxygen by facemask, and ventilation and resuscitation if their breathing stops.

What else can I do?

Ensure your child is fully immunised.

WHAT TO DO IN AN EMERGENCY

If your baby stops breathing after a coughing spasm, try to stimulate respiration by gentle physical contact. At the same time get urgent medical help. Clear the mouth of any vomit to prevent it being inhaled. If there is no response start doing mouth-to-mouth resuscitation.

CHAPTER 10

ACCIDENT PREVENTION AND FIRST AID

MOST accidents are preventable, but the sad statistics show that each year in the UK 1 million children – from newborn babies to 15-year-olds – visit hospital because of an accident that occurred at home. Of these, 600,000 are in the 0-4-year-age group.

Accidents that happen outside the home account for another 1.4 million injuries per year, with 86 per cent of these occurring in the over-4s.

In 1995 there were 185 fatalities from accidents in the home (England and Wales): 84 as a result of burns; 33 from suffocation or choking; 21 by drowning; 17 from falls; 11 from being struck by an object; 10 by poisoning; and 9 others. Outside the home, the main cause of death was from road accidents, totalling 306: 54 per cent affecting pedestrians, 30 per cent those in a vehicle and 16 per cent on a bicycle.

Safety in the home

To try to prevent your own child becoming part of those statistics, you must ensure that your home is as safe as it can be from the moment the baby is born. As he or she grows and understands more, you can teach safety skills and rules.

Young babies
Many young babies end up at the doctor's surgery or the hospital having suffered a head injury after falling off a surface, perhaps

during a nappy change. All but the most minor of head injuries should be checked by a doctor. Signs to look out for initially are a loss of consciousness, vomiting and failure to move one or more limbs, and, over the next 24 to 48 hours, undue drowsiness, further vomiting or refusal to feed. After 48 hours the danger period is likely to have passed. If any symptoms persist or you are still worried, don't hesitate to go back again for a further check. See also **Head injuries** below.

The other main danger at this age is the bath. A baby should never be left unattended as it is possible to drown in only a few inches of water. Also, take care with the temperature of the water, and remember that an older sibling could easily turn on the hot tap and then be unable to turn it off. It is recommended that the hot water thermostat is turned down to 54°C (130°F). See also **Drowning** below.

Crawling babies

Once a baby begins to crawl many new dangers appear. Put all your preventative measures into effect long before this stage so that you get used to working round them.

- Protect fires with fireguards.
- Position electrical wires and cables out of reach, and protect sockets with special plastic covers.
- An iron presents a very real danger for an inquisitive child – don't leave a child and the iron unattended in the same room.
- Move small, sharp (or valuable) objects out of reach.
- Fit stairgates at both the bottom and the top of stairs.
- Small toys, usually belonging to an older sibling, could be swallowed or inhaled by a small child. Throw any broken toys away.
- Don't allow the child to eat foods such as peanuts in case of choking.
- Lock medicines out of sight and out of reach in a cabinet. Remember, often the simplest medicines such as paracetamol or aspirin are the most dangerous in overdose.
- Family pets, particularly cats and dogs, should be regarded as a potential danger to a baby. Don't leave your baby unattended in the presence of the pet – even a docile animal can turn nasty.

Toddlers

As the baby learns to walk further dangers need to be considered.

- Lock any windows which the child could open and climb through.
- Protect glass panels in doors or furniture, if they are not made of safety glass, by wooden panels. Glass can be covered with safety film (cling film) which will hold broken pieces of glass in place if they are accidentally broken.
- Attach special corner protectors to any low sharp corners on furniture.
- Replace any worn parts of carpets and avoid using loose rugs in corridors, especially on top of smooth fitted floorcoverings.
- Never dry clothes on airers standing close to any fire, or draped over a convector heater.

The kitchen

- Keep a fire blanket near the cooker.
- Cook at the back of the hob, and turn saucepan handles to the back; use a safety rail around the top of the cooker
- Don't leave a chip pan to heat up unattended.
- Never put a tea-towel over the hob.
- Avoid dangling flexes: use short curly flex where appropriate.
- Keep bleach and household cleaners etc. securely locked in cupboards or out of reach.
- Fit child locks to cupboards the child can reach easily.
- Check that your oven door does not become too hot when in use. There may be a problem with older types of cookers.
- Keep the oven door closed.
- Keep the floor clean and dry.
- Don't leave knives lying around.
- Never lift a hot pan and carry a child at the same time.

The garage
The garage is often the dumping ground for a whole host of belongings, many of them dangerous to a child – heavy objects, sharp tools, electricity cables. Keep any chemicals such as weed-killer, antifreeze etc. out of reach, preferably in childproof bottles.

The garden

- Ponds and streams are a drowning hazard for a young child and need to be made safe. Cover a pond or even drain it, until your child is older.

- Keep a constant eye on children using a paddling pool.
- Greenhouse glass can easily be broken – if possible, put up some kind of barrier such as wooden trellis.
- The garden may contain poisonous plants and berries. Teach your child never to put any part of a plant in the mouth unless you have said that it is all right to eat it.
- The garden can be an escape route into the outside world for a child – make sure gates and fences are secure.
- Keep all hard surfaces – patios, paths, steps etc. – in good condition.
- Keep all obstacles to a minimum, clearing up hoses, tools and so on as soon as you have finished with them.
- Cover all canes that are supporting plants with rubber or plastic caps, or use upturned yoghurt pots, to protect eyes.
- Make sure that all play equipment is secure.
- Avoid free-standing ornaments such as bird baths – they are at just the right height to injure a child who is not looking where he or she is going.
- Supervise a barbecue or bonfire at all times.
- Follow the firework code.

First aid

It is important for parents and carers to know what to do if a child has an accident. In an emergency, simple first aid can assist recovery while you are waiting for medical help; for relatively minor injuries, you can help the child (and yourself) to keep calm if you know what to do.

If you are unsure about the nature of an injury or are worrying whether to take your child to the accident and emergency department at the hospital or your GP, that is probably reason enough for taking the child for examination. If there is an obvious problem, particularly if you suspect a fracture, the accident and emergency department would be your first port of call. If a few days have elapsed since the injury and you are still worried, take your child to your GP. If you are in an unfamiliar place, say on holiday, take the child to the local accident and emergency department, although a local GP would also be able to see the child as a temporary patient.

Bites and stings

Insects and animals do not usually attack children unless provoked. Teach your child not to tease animals.

Animal bites

An animal bite is usually a significant injury and always merits medical attention. One of the reasons for this is that animals (like humans) can carry bugs in their mouth which are deposited at the site of the bite. Ultimately, this can lead to infections – some of them can be nasty.

For a superficial bite, clean the wound by dousing it with running water for five minutes and dry it by patting it with a clean towel or garment. Cover the bite with a dry dressing and seek medical advice either from your own doctor or the local accident and emergency department.

For a more serious bite, apply pressure to the wound with a clean dressing, keeping the injured part of the body raised up. Then cover the wound with a pad and bandage it in place. Take the child to the accident and emergency department.

Insect stings

A bee leaves its sting embedded within the skin while a wasp does not. If you can see the sting remove it with tweezers as close to the skin as possible. Place a cold compress on the area to reduce pain and swelling. Later, apply some antiseptic to the site.

If the child has been stung in the mouth take him or her to the accident and emergency department for a check-up, as any swelling can obstruct the airway and cause breathing difficulties. A good first-aid measure on the way to hospital is to get the child to suck on ice cubes to help reduce the swelling.

Very rarely, a severe and life-threatening allergic reaction to an insect sting can occur. The child very quickly becomes ill and may even lose consciousness in a short period of time. The face may swell up and the eyes go puffy, and the child may have difficulty breathing; the pulse rate may also go up. This is called an anaphylactic reaction (see page 43 for further information). Dial 999 straight away as this can be a grave emergency.

Broken bones

Sometimes it is obvious if there is a fracture, but often you can tell only with an x-ray: sprains and strains can be just as painful as a fracture and can cause as much tenderness and swelling.

- Start by checking the child's breathing and pulse in case you need to resuscitate him or her (see page 264).
- Be alert for signs of shock, such as cold, clammy skin, rapid shallow breathing, weak pulse or fainting. To treat shock, lie the child down, loosen tight clothing, raise and support the legs, and keep him or her warm.
- Don't move a suspected broken arm or leg until it has been checked by a doctor.
- To make a splint, use a straight, rigid object (e.g. a stick or a broom handle); it should be longer than the bone and padded with soft material such as clothing or a blanket.
- Tie the padded splint to the injured limb, but not too tightly. Check regularly that the fingers or toes are not going blue.
- Put a splinted arm into a sling.
- In case a general anaesthetic is needed, do not give food or drink to the child.
- Move the child only if it is really necessary, and only after the injury has been splinted.

One special fracture to be aware of in young children is a greenstick fracture. This is more of a buckling in a bone than a clean break. Usually, such fractures are diagnosed by an x-ray and will heal by themselves with no surgical intervention.

Bruising and soft tissue injuries

A bruise is caused by the seeping out of blood from injured blood vessels. In itself, bruising represents an injury to the soft tissues such as muscles or ligaments, but remember that it can also be a sign of a more serious injury such as a fracture.

To reduce bruising and painful swelling to an injured part, cool it for about 10-15 minutes – a bag of frozen peas with a damp tea-towel acting as a bandage round both the peas and the injury is ideal (do not put the ice in direct contact with the skin). This works by reducing the flow of blood to the injury. Make sure that the compression is not too tight, remembering to allow for a degree of swelling when applying the bandage. First-aid measures will not completely abolish the swelling.

Burns and scalds

- Remove any clothing that has been immersed in hot fat, boiling water or caustic chemicals, unless it has already stuck to the skin. Don't take off cooled, dry burnt clothes, as this could introduce infection.
- Flood the burnt or scalded area gently with cold water for ten minutes (water from a pond or stream is better than nothing) or another cold liquid if water is not available, such as beer, milk or wine.
- Carefully remove jewellery and any constricting clothing before the injured area swells.
- Once cooled, the burn should be protected by a clean covering which has no hairs or filaments, such as cotton (not cotton wool), cling-wrap, or a plastic bag.
- Take the child to hospital.

If the child is in shock, lay him or her down, protecting the damaged area from contact with the ground, with the legs slightly raised and head turned to one side to prevent choking; then call for emergency help, give sips of water, and loosen any tight clothing.

Do not use an adhesive dressing, plaster or any fluffy material such as cotton wool.
Do not apply any butter, grease, oil, lotion etc.
Do not burst any blisters or remove loose skin as this will increase the risk of infection.

HOW TO STOP CLOTHES BURNING

- Stop the child panicking or running around.
- Lie the child on the ground.
- Wrap him or her tightly in a blanket, coat or any other non-flammable material.
- Roll the child over until the flames have been smothered.
- If water is available, lay the child down, burning side uppermost; then put out the flames by dousing the area with water.

Cuts and wounds

A lot of first aid is plain common sense but often that can go out of the window when we are dealing with a child who has suddenly been injured. A small blood loss can look more than it actually is. Usually the bleeding stops itself but occasionally it may not.

- If possible first wash your hands and wear disposable gloves if these are readily available.
- *Do not* attempt to dislodge any deeply embedded object.
- Remove any *loose* dirt or gravel etc.
- Rinse under cold water.
- Gently clean the surrounding area, using a damp clean cloth or an antiseptic wipe, wiping *away* from the wound.
- If dirt or grit remains in a graze, use a clean soft nail brush, ideally under cold running water.
- Pat the area dry with a clean, non-fluffy cloth.
- Cover a small wound with a plaster; use a sterile gauze pad and a bandage or plaster to cover larger cuts or grazes.

If blood continues to flow, apply pressure directly over the injured area, unless an object is embedded in it.

- Lie the child down, with legs slightly raised. If it is the arm that is injured raise that too.
- Press a clean cloth firmly over the wound, so that the wound edges are held together.
- Maintain this pressure continuously by bandaging a pad tightly over the cloth.
- If blood soaks through the pad, bandage another one over the top. *Do not* remove the original bandage and pad.
- You may be able to reduce the bleeding by applying a bag of frozen peas on top of the bandage.

If an object is embedded in the skin:

- Loosely drape a clean cloth over the wound and the object.
- Build up pads of gauze around the wound until they are above the height of the object.
- Secure the pads with a firmly applied bandage, without bandaging over the object itself.
- Seek medical help.

Also seek medical help if:

- Bleeding is severe or does not stop after 20 minutes.
- Shock develops: pallor, dizziness, extreme thirst, cold and clammy skin, weak pulse and rapid shallow breathing.
- The wound is a puncture injury e.g. from a nail.
- The cut is dirty, jagged or gaping.

Drowning

Even though it is stating the obvious, young children, particularly those who have just learnt to walk, should never be left near water unattended, even for just a few moments – a bath, an ornamental pond in the garden, or a stream or canal near a play area can be lethal. Older children and teenagers are also at risk of drowning when they do not fully appreciate the potential hazards. As soon as your child is old enough, teach him or her to be proficient swimmers and to have a healthy respect for all water hazards.

If a child does fall in water, get him out and keep the head lower than the body. If he is unconscious, check that he is breathing and place him in the recovery position – see page 266. (See 'cardio-pulmonary resuscitation' on pages 265 and 268 if he is not breathing.) Take the child to hospital, even if he seems recovered, in case he has inhaled water.

Electric shock

Impress on your child the importance of never playing with sockets, wires or flex, and of never bringing water into contact with an electrical appliance.

If your child has been in an electrical accident:

- Switch off the current at the mains.
- If you cannot do this, stand on dry material such as wood or a book, and use a broom handle or chair leg to push the child away from the source of the electricity.
- *Do not* touch the child, but pull him right away by wrapping a dry cloth or towel round his legs.
- Call for emergency help.

Foreign bodies

An insect in the ear may be washed out by pouring water gently into the ear; one in the eye may be removed with the corner of a clean handkerchief or cloth. If you have any difficulty removing an object from the eye, ear or nose, take the child to hospital.

If the child has swallowed an object, find out what is: something small like a plum stone or a small coin will eventually pass through the body, but if the object was large or sharp, don't give the child anything to eat or drink and take him to hospital.

Choking

If something has got caught in the larynx (voice box), the child may cough, become distressed and have obvious difficulty in breathing. The procedures differ according to whether you are dealing with a baby or a child. In either case, do not feel blindly down the throat, and if at any time the obstruction clears or the infant becomes unconscious begin resuscitation (see page 264).

Baby

- Lay the baby face down along your forearm, keeping his head low.
- Give up to five sharp slaps on the back.
- Turn the baby face up on your arm or lap.
- Check the mouth and remove anything obvious with one finger, without touching the baby's throat.
- If the back slaps fail to work, place two fingertips on the lower half of the baby's breastbone, one finger's breadth below the nipples.
- Give up to five sharp thrusts into the chest, and check the mouth again.
- Repeat the entire sequence three times. If the obstruction has not cleared, take the baby with you to the phone to dial for an ambulance.
- Keep repeating the steps until help arrives.

Child

- With the child standing, bend him forwards.

- Give up to five sharp slaps between his shoulders with one hand.
- Check his mouth and take out any obvious obstruction.
- If the back slaps fail, stand or kneel behind the child.
- With one hand make a fist and place it against his lower breast-bone.
- Grasp the hand with the other hand and press into the chest with a sharp inward thrust up to five times, at a rate of about one every three seconds.
- Check the mouth again; if choking persists, give up to five back slaps as before.
- Check the mouth again and if necessary go to the next step.
- Make a fist and place it against the child's central upper abdomen, lower than the previous position.
- Grasp your fist with your other hand and press with a sharp inward thrust up to five times.
- Check the mouth once more; then dial for an ambulance if necessary.
- Keep repeating the sequence of back slaps and chest and abdominal thrusts until help arrives.

Head injury

If the child is unconscious, get medical help immediately.

- Check the child is breathing, carefully move him into the recovery position (page 266). If any fluid is coming from the ear or nose, place a sterile dressing over the orifice and turn the head towards the injured side, but do not apply pressure or try to block the flow.
- If the child is not breathing and has no pulse, start resuscitating him – see page 264.
- *Do not* turn the child on to one side if you suspect a neck injury.
- Keep a close watch on the child until medical help arrives.
- If there is a cut on the scalp or face, the bleeding will be profuse. Try to stop the bleeding by applying constant pressure with a sterile dressing or clean cloth, but if there is a foreign body or fragment of bone in the wound, cover the area without pressing on it.

- If there is a bump on the head, apply an ice pack (or a bag of frozen peas wrapped in a cold wet tea-towel) to reduce the pain and swelling.

Heat exhaustion

Make the child lie down in a cool room, with his legs raised, and give him a cold drink.

Poisoning

Every household contains numerous poisonous substances. Keep all medicines, cleaning fluids, plant foods and so on out of reach and out of sight in childproof cupboards. Review your storage arrangements as the child gets older and smarter, and take any medicines that are out of date or redundant to the pharmacist for disposal. Never decant poisonous substances into bottles previously used for drink, for instance, or that look in any way appealing.

If the child has swallowed a poisonous substance:

- Give him frequent sips of water if he has swallowed a corrosive liquid such as bleach.
- If he is unconscious but breathing, put him in the recovery position (page 266). Check that the airway is clear of vomit and tilt the head back.
- If the child is not breathing apply cardio-pulmonary resuscitation (see page 265 and 268).
- *Do not* induce vomiting.
- For an inhaled poison, take the child into fresh air.
- Seek emergency help, taking any loose pills or suspect bottles with you; don't rely on your memory for names of medication that may have been swallowed.

Harmful/Irritant

Toxic/Very Toxic

Corrosive

Splinters

Clean round the area with warm water and soap. Pass the ends of a pair of tweezers (not a needle) through a match flame, and allow them to cool. Without wiping the sterilised tweezers, try to pull out the splinter at the same angle that it went into the skin, grabbing it as close as possible to the skin. When the splinter has come out squeeze the wound to make it bleed a little.

Take the child to the surgery if the splinter or part of it remains in the skin.

Sprains and strains

A sprain is a slight or partial tear in a ligament which is often found near a joint, while a strain is a muscle injury. Like bruising, these are soft tissue injuries.

THE RICE PROCEDURE FOR SPRAINS AND STRAINS

A good mnemonic for dealing with sprains is:

Rest the injured part
Apply Ice or a cold compress every ten to fifteen minutes (a pack of frozen peas wrapped in a wet teatowel is a good way to do this; do not put ice in direct contact with the skin)
Compress the injury with an elasticated stocking bandage. The bandage should extend well above and below the injury and should not be so tight as to cut off the circulation.
Elevate the injured part so that it is above the heart, if possible.

Sunburn

Prevention is better than cure: a wide range of sun creams is available. It is not just the short-term pain of sunburn that needs to be considered, but also the long-term damaging effects of the sun on the skin. Over-exposure to the sun without adequate protection is particularly harmful to children. Premature ageing of the skin and the possible risk of skin cancer (malignant melanoma) are the two main worries.

Sunburn itself is similar to an ordinary burn. Mild symptoms are redness and pain in the affected area, and sunburn is best treated by cooling with water or soothing after-sun lotions. More severe sunburn can cause blistering and peeling, and medical help should be sought.

Resuscitation for children

The techniques for resuscitating children differ according to their ages.

Babies under 12 months

- Check the baby's response by shaking him very gently.
- Lie the baby on his back on a flat surface and check the breathing for ten seconds by feeling any breath on your cheek and looking along the chest for signs of movement.
- If the baby is breathing and his pulse can be felt, put him into the **recovery position**: cradle him in your arms with his head tilted downwards. This prevents him from choking on his tongue or from inhaling vomit.

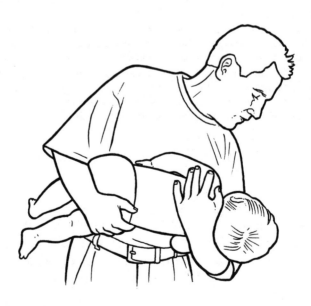

If the baby is *not* breathing:

- Lie him down on his back and carefully remove any *obvious* obstruction from the mouth.
- Seal your lips tightly around the mouth and nose, and breathe into the lungs.
- Give five breaths of mouth-to-mouth ventilation, aiming at one complete breath every three seconds.
- If there is no pulse or other sign of recovery, or if the pulse rate is below 60 per minute, apply **cardio-pulmonary resuscitation**: with the baby on his back, place the tips of two fingers on the lower breastbone, which is one finger's breadth below the inter-nipple line.
- Press down sharply at this point to a third of the depth of the chest. Do this five times quite fast (100 compressions per minute).

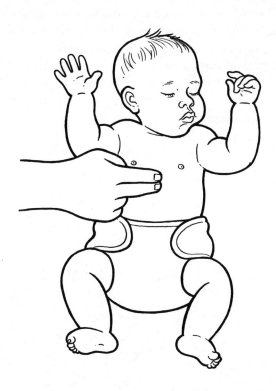

- Give one full breath of artificial ventilation as before; and then alternate giving five chest compressions and one breath of artificial ventilation.
- Follow the sequence for one minute before calling an ambulance; then continue until help arrives.

Children aged 1-7 years

- Check the child's response by shaking him very gently.
- Lie the child on his back on a flat surface and check the breathing for ten seconds by feeling any breath on your cheek and looking along the chest for signs of movement.
- If the child is breathing and his pulse is working, put him into the **recovery position**, as follows.
- With the child on his back, kneel beside him.
- Open his airway by gently tilting the head and lifting the chin. Straighten his legs.
- Tuck his hand that is nearest to you, the arm straight and palm upwards, under his upper thigh. Before turning him remove any fragile or bulky objects from his pockets.
- Bring the arm furthest from you across the chest, and hold the back of the hand against the child's nearest cheek. With your other hand, pull up the far leg just above the knee, keeping the foot flat on the ground.

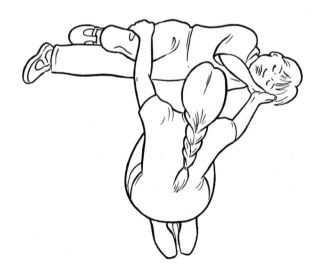

- Keeping the child's hand pressed against his cheek, pull on the upper leg to roll him towards you and on to his side.

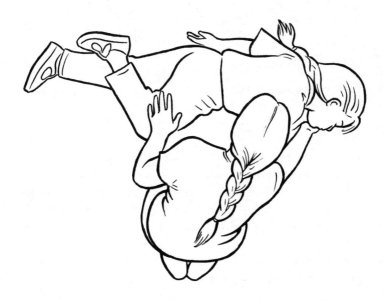

- Use your knees to support the child so that he is prevented from rolling too far forwards.
- Tilt the head back to ensure the airway remains open. If necessary, adjust the hand under the cheek.
- Adjust the upper leg, if necessary, so that both the hip and the knee are both at right angles.
- Adjust the lower arm so that the child is not lying on it. Make sure that his hand is still positioned with the palm facing upwards.

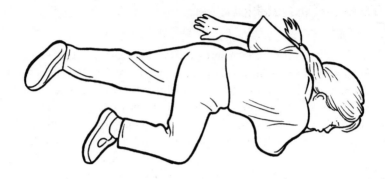

- Call an ambulance; and continue to monitor the breathing and pulse until help arrives.

If the child is *not* breathing:

- Lie him down on his back and carefully remove any *obvious* obstruction from the mouth.
- Pinch his nostrils closed. Seal your lips tightly around the mouth, and breathe into the lungs until the chest rises.
- Give five breaths of mouth-to-mouth ventilation, allowing about two seconds for inflation.
- If there is no pulse or other sign of recovery apply **cardio-pulmonary resuscitation**: with the child on his back, place the heel of one of your hands where the ribs meet at the breastbone.
- Press down sharply at this point to a third of the depth of the chest. Do this five times quite fast.
- Give one full breath of artificial ventilation as before; and then alternate giving five chest compressions and one breath of artificial ventilation.
- Follow the sequence for one minute before calling an ambulance; then continue until help arrives.

Children over eight years
Follow the instructions as for a child up to the age of seven, but give two full breaths at a time, and use the heels of both your hands, fingers interlocking, to give 15 chest compressions at a time. Alternate these two actions until help arrives.

A home first-aid kit

All parents know only too well that their child will get into a scrape at some point and sustain a minor injury, so it is a good idea to keep a first-aid kit in the house as well as the car. You can buy reasonably stocked first-aid kits but you can cut the cost of these and have a more comprehensive version by making one up for yourself. The kit should be housed in a well-marked container and placed in a prominent and accessible site (although out of reach to young hands).

Inspect the kit every year and check the contents, particularly medicines, to see that they have not gone beyond their use-by date. The following items make up a basic household first-aid kit; you may need to add certain items if members of your family have particular needs.

The best first-aid kit is one you put together yourself:

- cotton bandages/contour bandages – one 5cm, one 7.5cm wide
- crêpe bandages – one 5cm, one 7.5cm wide
- eye pad (an extra non-adhesive wound dressing can be used instead, but it needs to be large enough to cover the whole eye area)
- gauze swabs – at least four
- plasters – 15-20 individually wrapped, some waterproof
- safety pins
- strong scissors (strong enough to cut through fabric)
- surgical tape (if dressings are not adhesive)
- triangular bandage
- wound dressings, both medium and large sizes
- eye bath

To make up a kit for the **car**, also include alcohol-free antiseptic wipes, a large wound dressing, latex gloves to protect yourself or the injured person from infection in case of blood spillages, a triangular bandage and a foil blanket to keep the injured person warm.

A home medicine cupboard

Although you cannot make provision for every eventuality, it is worth keeping a range of preparations in your medicine cupboard to treat common minor ailments. Remember that the main danger presented by most medicines is taking them in overdose, and that the ones most easily available, such as paracetamol, are the most dangerous. Always keep medicines, creams and so on safely out of reach and if possible locked away, and remind guests to be disciplined about keeping their personal medication out of sight and out of reach. If you suspect that your child has taken an overdose seek medical help immediately.

Make a point of checking all these preparations regularly and asking your pharmacist to dispose of any that are past their use-by date or are leaking or damaged in some way.

For every medicine, double-check the dosage for your child's age group before you give it to him or her, and never let your child take a medicine without your supervision.

Pain relief and fever

Paracetamol (Calpol) can be used as a painkiller and will also help to reduce a fever. The liquid form is probably more easily taken by younger children, while the soluble tablet form may be preferred by older children.

Ibuprofen (Junifen) is an alternative to paracetamol: as it has greater anti-inflammatory properties it may be better for treating pain caused by injury.

Aspirin should not be given to children under 12 years because of the risk of Reye's Syndrome, a rare but serious reaction to the drug.

Antihistamines

Promethazine (Phenergan) or chlorpheniramine (Piriton) are two sedative antihistamines which are useful for treating the itch of eczema or chickenpox. In fact, they are often used purely for their sedative effects on young children. Allergic conditions such as hay fever tend to be treated with newer less sedative antihistamines.

Coughs and colds

Babies may be bothered by a blocked or runny nose and their feeding may be affected, but the condition is often best left untreated. For older infants and children, nasal decongestants, usually in the form of drops such as Children's formula Otrivine nasal drops, may help.

A wide range of cough medicines is available over the counter – ask your pharmacist for advice. You may wish to choose a preparation that is sugar-free.

Because most coughs and colds are caused by viruses, antibiotics are ineffective.

Teething

When babies are unsettled and crying, teething is usually high on the list of possible causes. The gums can become painful as the teeth approach the surface and break through. Paracetamol liquid (Calpol) can help with relieving pain.

Tummy upsets

These usually start with vomiting, diarrhoea or both. The most useful action you can take is to give your child plenty of drinks, such as weak fruit juice or squash. If you are breastfeeding, don't stop. Solutions such as Dioralyte, Electrolade and Rehidrat, come in sachets of various flavours, which when mixed with the correct amount of water produce a drink containing the correct concentration of salts and minerals to correct dehydration.

Colic, nappy rash and eczema

The treatment of these conditions is covered on page 28 (colic), page 35–6 (nappy rash) and page 184 (eczema).

ADDRESSES

Action for Victims of Medical Accidents
Bank Chambers
1 London Road
Forest Hill
London SE23 3TP
0181-291 2793

Anthony Nolan Bone Marrow Trust
Unit 2
Heathgate Buildings
75-87 Agincourt Road
London NW3 2NT
0171-284 1234

Association of Breastfeeding Mothers
PO Box 441
St Albans
Herts AL4 0AS
0181-778 4769

Association for Children with Heart Disorders
26 Elizabeth Drive
Helmshore
Rossendale
Lancs BB4 4JB
(01706) 213632

Association of Community Health Councils for England & Wales
30 Drayton Pk
London N5 1PB
0171-609 8405

Association for Post-Natal Illness
25 Jerdan Place
London SW6 1BE
0171-386 0868

Association for Spina Bifida and Hydrocephalus
ASBAH House
42 Park Road
Peterborough
Cambs PE1 2UQ
(01733) 555988

British Diabetic Association
10 Queen Anne Street
London W1M 0BD
0171-323 1531

British Epilepsy Association
Anstey House
40 Hanover Square
Leeds
W Yorks LS3 1BE
Helpline: (0800) 309030

Cleft Lip and Palate Association
134 Buckingham Palace Road
London SW1W 9SA
0171-824 8110

Coeliac Society
PO Box 220
High Wycombe
Bucks HP11 2HY
(01494) 437278

Cot death helpline
see Foundation for the Study of
Infant Deaths

CRY-SIS
BM CRY-SIS
London WC1N 3XX
24-hour helpline: 0171-404 5011

Cystic Fibrosis Trust
11 London Road
Bromley
Kent BR1 1BY
0181-464 7211

Down's Syndrome Association
155 Mitcham Road
London SW17 9PG
0181-682 4001

Dyslexia Institute
133 Gresham Road
Staines
Middx TW18 2AJ
(01784) 463851

**Foundation for the Study of
Infant Deaths**
14 Halkin Street
London SW1X 7DP
0171-235 0965
Cot death helpline (24-hour service):
0171-235 1721

Fragile X Society
53 Winchelsea Lane
Hastings
East Sussex TN35 4LG
(01424) 813147

General Dental Council
37 Wimpole Street
London W1M 8DQ
0171-486 2171

General Medical Council
178 Great Portland Street
London W1N 6JE
0171-580 7642

Health Service Ombudsman
11–14th floor
Millbank Tower
Millbank
London SW1P 4QP
0171-217 4051
Information line on NHS com-
plaints procedure: (0800) 665544

**La Leche League of Great
Britain**
BM 3424
London WC1N 3XX
0171-242 1278

National Asthma Campaign
Providence House
Providence Place
London N1 0NT
0171-226 2260

National Autistic Society
393 City Road
London EC1V 1NE
0171-833 2299

National Childbirth Trust
Alexandra House
Oldham Terrace
London W3 6NH
0181-992 8637

National Deaf Children's Society
15 Dufferin Street
London EC1Y 8PD
0171-250 0123

National Eczema Society
163 Eversholt Street
London NW1 1BU
0171-388 4097
Helpline: 0171-388 4800

NHS Confederation
26 Chapter Street
London SW1P 4ND
0171-233 7388

National Meningitis Trust
Fern House, Bath Road
Stroud
Gloucs GL5 3TJ
(01453) 751738
Helpline: (0345) 538118

National Society for the Prevention of Cruelty to Children
42 Curtain Road
London EC2A 3NH
0171-825 2500
24-hour helpline: (0800) 800500

Parents At Work
45 Beech Street
London EC2Y 8AD
0171-628 3565
Information line: 0171-628 3578
Special needs helpline: 0171-588 0802

Patients Association
PO Box 935
Harrow
Middx HA1 3YJ
0171-242 3460

Scope (formerly the Spastics Society)
12 Park Crescent
London W1N 4EQ
0171-636 5020
Helpline: (0800) 626216

UK Central Council for Nursing, Midwifery and Health Visiting
23 Portland Place
London W1N 4JT
0171-637 7181

Young Arthritis Care
18 Stephenson Way
London NW1 2HD
0171-916 1500

INDEX

Page numbers in **bold** indicate where a subject is dealt with in more detail.

abdominal pain 193, 194, 237
  see also appendicitis
accident prevention 56, **251–4**
  crawling babies 252
  electrical safety 252
  in the garden 253–4
  in the home 251–3
  kitchen safety 253
  toddlers 252–3
  young babies 251–2
acupressure 14
acupuncture 14, 151, 203
adolescents 119, 139
aggressive tendencies 119
AIDS 12
allergens 146
allergies 84, 94, 105, **146–8**
  see also cows' milk allergy;
    eczema; hay fever; mercury
    allergy
amniocentesis **14**, 181
anaemia 157, 162, 211, 237
  see also thalassaemia
anal fissures 167, 168
anaphylaxis **43**, 106, 146, 148, 255
anorexia nervosa 121
antenatal screening 13–14, 22, 30
anti-convulsants 33
anti-depressants 89
anti-social behaviour 117, **119–20**
antibiotics 232, 271
antihistamines 147, 185, 202, 270
anxiety 14, 119, 203
aphthous ulcers 131
appendicitis **148–9**, 193

appetite loss 119, 157, 172, 204, 231, 245
aromatherapy 14, 37
arthritis **149–51**, 193, 205, 215, 216, 224
aspirin 203, 270
asthma 104, 105, 146, **151–5**, 201, 202, 230
  emergency action 155
  inhalers 153, 154
  peak flows 153, 154, 155
  steroids 153–4
  symptoms 152
atopic eczema 184
attention deficit disorder 117
autism 69, **115–16**

bathroom safety 252
BCG vaccine 46, 52, 209
bed-sharing 40
bedwetting 56, **79–80**, 176
behavioural and emotional problems 56, 105, **109–22**
  anti-social behaviour 117, **119–20**
  assessment 110
  autism 69, **115–16**
  child neglect and abuse 17, **121–2**
  consistency in dealing with 71, 85, 86
  delayed development 111
  dyslexia 113–15
  eating disorders 121
  factors at the root of 109–10
  hyperactivity 116–18

infants and younger children
110–18
new baby in the family 112–13
school refusal 119, **120**
schoolchildren 118–22
sibling jealousy 56, 113
speech problems 111–12
tackling 110
see also crying; Fragile X
Syndrome; sleep problems;
temper tantrums; toilet training
bilirubin 21, 204
birthmarks 22
birth weight 18, 29, 56, 57, **91**
bites and stings 255
bladder control *see* toilet training
bleeding and bruising 204, 211
blink reflex 62
blisters *see* chickenpox; hand, foot
and mouth disease; impetigo
blood tests 14, 106, 138
'blue babies' 25, 164
body lice 213, 214
body temperature 17, 78, 82, 192
bone cancer *see* Ewing's sarcoma;
osteosarcoma
bone infections 49
bone marrow damage 51
bone marrow transplant 212–13
bottle decay 125
bottle-feeding **95–8**
additional water and juices 98
changing from breast-feeding to
89–90
feeder cups 97
full-fat cows' milk, introducing
97–8
quantities 96–7
solids in bottles 102
vitamin supplements 97
see also formula milks
bowel obstructions 26
bowel problems 26–7
see also coeliac disease;
constipation; diarrhoea;
gastro-enteritis

brain damage 10, 12, 17, 22, 44, 48,
50, 51, 122, 203
see also cerebral palsy
brain scans 156, 190
brain tumours **156**, 203
breast-feeding **92–5**
allergies and 105
and baby's weight gain 59
benefits of breast milk **92**, 105
changing to bottle-feeding 89–90
demand feeding 93
diet while 94
duration 94–5
expressing breast milk 92, 93
milk flow 93
successful breast-feeding 92–3
'top-up' feeds 93
vegetarian mothers 106
and vitamin supplements 95
working mothers 89–90
breath-holding attacks **86–7**, 187
breathing, noisy 28, 168–9
breathing problems
emergency action 169, 187
first-year problems 27–8
premature babies 18
see also asthma; croup; diphtheria;
epiglottitis
breathlessness *see* wheezing and
breathlessness
breech babies 20
bribery 86
brittle nails 234
broken bones 256
broken and dysfunctional homes 119
bronchiectasis 231
bronchiolitis 28
bronchitis 230–1
bruising and soft tissue injuries 256–7
bulimia nervosa 121
bullying 120
burns and scalds 257
'Buzzer' (bedwetting detector pad) 80

caffeine intake 11, 94
calamine lotion 147, 160

calculus 131–2
Calpol 270, 271
cancer 56, **155–60**
    bone cancer 158–9
    brain tumours **156**, 203
    Ewing's sarcoma 159
    leukaemia 161, 181, 204, **211–13**
    malignant melanoma **158**, 263
    neuroblastoma 157–8
    osteosarcoma 158–9
    retinoblastoma 156–7
    of the testicles 38, 240
    Wilm's tumour 157
cancer screening 56
candidiasis 35
carbamazepine 190
caries 123
cataracts 19, 51
catarrh 27, 182–3, 217, 230
centile charts 58–9
cerebral palsy 17, **25–6**, 69, 215
chest infections *see* respiratory tract
        infections
chickenpox 44, **160–1**, 212
Child Health Surveillance
        Programme 53, 54
child neglect and abuse 17, **121–2**
child psychiatrists 110, 119
childbirth *see* labour and delivery
Chinese herbal medicines 185–6
chlorpheniramine 270
choking 260–1
cholesterol 198
chorionic villus biopsy **14**, 181
circumcision 227, **228**
cleft lip and palate **23–4**, 184
clingy behaviour 64
club foot 20–1
clumsiness 113, 114
coeliac disease 92, 105, 111, **161–2**
colds 27, 193, 230, 249, 270–1
colic **28–9**, 82, 94, **101**
colitis 193
colostrum 92
community dental service 128
Community Health Councils 140

community health doctors 53
community psychiatric nurses 89
complaints
    about dental treatment 129
    about health care 139–43, 145
    compensation 140, **143**, 145
complementary therapy
    acupressure 14
    acupuncture 14, 151, 203
    aromatherapy 14, 37
    Chinese herbal medicines 185–6
    GP attitudes to 135
    herbal medicine 14, 45, 80, 151,
        185, 246
    homeopathy 37, 78, 80, 101, 151,
        154, 185
    hypnosis 14
    massage 14, 78, 83
    relaxation therapy 154–5
    yoga 154–5
computerised tomography 156
computers and computer games 73
concentration, poor 113, 114
concussion 203
congenital abnormalities 13, **22–6**
congenital heart disease 162–4, 181
congenital hernia 206
conjunctivitis 36, 146, **165–6**
symptoms 165
consistency in dealing with children
        71, 85, 86
constipation 56, 81, 100, **166–8**
contraception 56
controlled crying technique 75–6, 78
convergent squint 34
convulsions *see* epilepsy, febrile
        convulsions
cot death 17, **39–41**, 56
cot mattresses 40
cough medicines 27–8, 232, 271
coughing 27–8, 152, 172, 183, 193,
        194, 217, 230, 231, 270–1
    see also asthma; bronchitis; cystic
        fibrosis; measles; whooping
        cough
cows' milk 95, **97–8**, 104, 107

cows' milk allergy 94, 101, 105, 147, 197
cranial osteopathy 74, 101, 182
crawling/walking 55, 63, 65, 66
creative play 71
Crohn's disease 92
croup 28, **168–9**, 193
CRY-SIS 84
crying 61, 62, 78, **81–4**
    controlled crying technique 75–6, 78
    coping with 82–4
    reasons for 81–2
CT scans 156, 157
cuts and wounds 258–9
cyanosis 31
cystic fibrosis 21, 30, 111, **170–2**, 198
cytomegalovirus 12, 173

deafness 12, 22, 33, 50, 51, 111, **172–5**, 218, 224
    conductive deafness 173
    sensorineural deafness 173
decongestants 147, 270
dehydration 27, 48, 168, 169, 193, 196
dementia 181
dental abscesses 132
dental problems **129–32**
    acid erosion 130–1
    dental injuries 130
    gum disease 123, **131–2**
    mouth ulcers 131
    orthodontics 129–30
    thrush 131
    toothache 132
dental x-rays 127–8
dentistry 127–9, 163
dento-facial orthopaedics 130
depression 119
dermatitis 35, 147, 184
destructive behaviour 119
developmental *see* growth and development
dexamphetamine 118
diabetes 170, **175–7**
diaphragmatic hernia 206–7

diarrhoea 27, 30, 37, 56, 57, 105, 167, 178, 193, 204, 217, 218
    blood in 196–7
    see also constipation; gastro-enteritis; toddler's diarrhoea
diazepam 32
diet and nutrition 56, **91–108**
    while breast-feeding 94
    children's nutritional requirements 107
    deficiencies 104
    dietary deficiencies 104
    foods to avoid 99–100
    gluten-free diet 162
    good meals guide 103
    healthy eating principles 107–8
    in pregnancy 11
    problems 100–6
    solid foods 98–9, 104, 107
    vegan diet 96, **107**
    vegetarian diets 96, **106–7**
    vitamin supplements 95, 97, 104
    see also food allergies; weight
dimethicone 29
Dioralyte 196, 271
diphtheria 45, 46, 47, **178–80**, 243
discipline 86, 109
disclosing tablets 124
distraction test 67–8
divergent squint 34
DNA 13
Down's Syndrome 13, 14, 69, **180–2**, 198, 211
dressing 65
drooling 37
drowning 259
drowsiness 161, 193, 203, 220
dummies 78, 83, 100, 125
dyslexia 113–15
dysuria 245

ear drum, perforated 173, 183
ear infections 24, 27, 28, 174, **182–4**, 193, 194, 218
    otitis externa 183
    otitis media 182–3

see also glue ear
earache *see* ear infections
earwax, excess 173, 174
eating disorders 121
eczema 35, 101, 104, 105, 146, 147,
     152, 183, **184–6**, 202, 211
  atopic eczema 184
  dermatitis 35, 147, 184
  seborrhoeic eczema 184
eggs 104, 106
electric shock 259
electro-encephalogram (EEG) 190
Electrolade 196, 271
emollients (skin moisturisers) 185
emotional abuse 110
emotional deprivation 111
encephalitis 32, 44, 50, 161, 203, 218,
     219
encopresis 81
endocarditis 163, 164
enema 168
epiglottitis 45, 169, **186–7**
epilepsy 12, 26, 32, 87, 116, **187–91**
  first aid 189
  focal epilepsy 188
  grand mal epilepsy 188
  infantile spasms 188
  petit mal 188
  temporal lobe epilepsy 188
Ewing's sarcoma 159
exercise
  children 73–4
  during pregnancy 11
eye drops 166
eye muscle exercises 35
eye patches 35
eye problems
  cataracts 19, 51
  conjunctivitis 36, 146, **165–6**
  retinoblastoma 156–7
eyes
  discharge from 165, 217
  itchy and swollen 165, 201

facial swelling *see* mumps
failure to thrive 25, **29–31**, 105, **111**,
     162, 164
fainting 191–2
family doctors *see* GPs
family life, children and 87–8
febrile convulsions **31–3**, 190, 217
  emergency action 32
  immunisation and **43–4**, 51
feeder cups 97, 100
feeding
  baby feeding self 65, 67
  regurgitation of feeds 26, 30,
     101–2
  see also bottle feeding; breast-
     feeding; diet and nutrition;
     weaning
feeding difficulties 30, 55
  babies with cleft lip and palate
     23–4
  food refusal 102
  malabsorption 30
  poor feeding 100–1
  premature babies 17
  see also colic
fertility, male 38, 50, 170, 225
fever 37, 51, 157, 168, **192–4**, 203,
     204, 217, 220, 221, 231, 245, 270
  see also chicken pox; meningitis;
     mumps
fibre 100
fingers and toes, extra or missing 20
first aid **254–71**
  bites and stings 255
  broken bones 256
  bruising and soft tissue injuries
     256–7
  burns and scalds 257
  choking 260–1
  cuts and wounds 258–9
  drowning 259
  electric shock 259
  foreign bodies 260
  head injuries 251–2, **261–2**
  heat exhaustion 262
  kit 269
  medicine cupboard 269–71
  poisoning 262

resuscitation 264–8
seeking professional help 254
shock 256, 257
splinters 263
sprains and strains (RICE
    procedure) 263
sunburn 263–4
first-year problems 26–39
fissure sealant 124–5
fits 31
    benign fits 32
    and faints, differences between
        192
    see also epilepsy; febrile
        convulsions
flossing 124
fluid retention 204
fluoride 125–6
fluorosis 126
focal epilepsy 188
Foetal Alcohol Syndrome 10
folic acid 11, 23
fontanelles 19, 222
food additives 118
food allergies 101, **104–6**, 105, 107,
        146, 147
    in babies 104–5
    cows' milk allergy 94, 101, 105,
        147, 197
    exclusion diet 106
    high-risk babies 104
    in later childhood 105–6
    testing for 106
foreign bodies 260
foreskin problems *see* penile and
    foreskin problems
formula milks 93, **95–7**
    casein-protein-predominant
        formulae 95, 96
    choosing 96
    follow-on formula 95, 96, 107
    low-allergy formula 104, 105
    nutritional content 107
    pre-term formulae 95, 96
    soya-based formula 105
    vegan infant formula 107

whey-protein-predominant
    formulae 95, 96
Fragile X Syndrome 194–5

gait, unsteady 203
gallstones 237
garage and garden, safety in the
    253–4
gastro-enteritis **26–7**, 30, 92, **195–7**
General Medical Council 140
genetic abnormalities 198–9
genetic counselling 181
genetic screening **13–14**, **198–9**
    amniocentesis **14**, 181
    chorionic villus biopsy **14**, 181
    triple or quadruple blood test 14
genital herpes 12
German measles *see* rubella
gingivitis 131–2
glands, swollen *see* glandular fever;
    mumps
glandular fever 205
glue ear 24, 173, 174, **199–200**
gluten-free cereals 105
goats' milk 99
gonorrhoea 12
GPs 53, 110, **133–7**, 254
    assessing the services available
        134–6
    changing your doctor 134
    complaints about 140, 141–2
    finding a doctor 133–4
    out-of-hours care 136
    referral to a specialist 137–8
    registering your new baby with
        133
    routine examinations 67–8
    taking a child to 136–7
grand mal epilepsy 188
grandparents 88
grasp reflex 60
grief 109
gripe-water 29, 101
grommets 200
growth and development
    average growth patterns 56–7

delayed development 109, 111, 194
18–24-month assessment 68
fine movements 59–60, 61, 65, 66, 62, 63
growth impairment 151
identifying problems 69
large body movements 59, 60, 62–3, 65, 66
measurement 57–9
newborn and first-year babies 60–4
'normal' development 60
'normal' growth 91
physical examinations 18–21, 67, 68
routine assessments 55, **67–9**
second year 65–6
third year 66–7
see also hearing; social behaviour; speech; vision
gum disease 123, **131–2**
gum shields 130
Guthrie test 21

haemophilia 225
Haemophilus influenzae 186, 187, 220, 221
hand, foot and mouth disease 200–1
hand movements 59–60, 61, 63, 65
hay fever 146, 152, 165, **201–2**
head circumference 57–8
head injuries 251–2, **261–2**
head lice 213, 214, 215
headaches 156, 193, **202–3**, 220
HEAF test 46
health records 54
Health Service Ombudsman 141–2
health visitors 53, **54–6**, 68, 135, 140
child health care 55–6
contact and frequency of visits 54–5
drop-in clinics 55
family health care 56
help with post-natal depression 88–9
hearing **33**, 55, 60

milestones 33, 111–12, 173
newborn and first-year babies 61, 62, 63
second year 65
tests 68
hearing aids 174
hearing problems 24, 33, 111–12
see also deafness
heart disease 12, **24–5**, 30, 49, 51, 56, 198
arteries, narrowing of 25
congenital heart disease **162–4**, 181
endocarditis 163, 164
hole in the heart 25, 163
symptoms 163–4
heart murmurs 19, **24–5**
heart tracing 24
heartburn 14
heat exhaustion 262
heel prick test 21
hepatitis 186, **204–6**
hepatitis A 204, 206
hepatitis B 205–6
herbal medicine 14, 45, 80, 151, 154, 185, 246
hernias 20, 26, 38, **206–7**
congenital hernia 206
diaphragmatic hernia 206–7
hiatus hernia 30
inguinal hernia 206, 207
strangulation 207
umbilical hernia 207
herpes virus 131
hiatus hernia 30
hip dislocations 20
HIV *see* Human Immunodeficiency Virus
hoarse voice 169
hole in the heart 25, 163
homeopathy 37, 78, 80, 101, 151, 154, 185
hospital treatment 137–9
complaints about 142
hospitals
accident and emergency units 137
educational provision in 139

hospital stays 138–9
outpatient clinics 138
Human Immunodeficiency Virus
(HIV) 56, **207–10**
hunger 81–2
hydrocephalus 23
hydrocortisone 185
hyperactivity 116–18
hyperkinetic disorder 117
hypos (hypoglycaemic attacks)
177
hypospadias 227–8

ibuprofen 193, 203, 270
ill health, chronic 109
immune system 42, 209, 211
immunisation **42–52**, 56, 193
    active immunisation 42
    BCG vaccine 46, 52, 209
    boosters 46, 217
    for children with compromised
        immune systems 46
    common concerns 43–5
    diseases, vaccines and vaccine risks
        47–52
    DTP vaccine 45
    haemophilus influenzae type b (Hib)
        45, **49–50**, 223
    MMR vaccine 44, **45–6**, 51
    passive immunisation 42
    pneumococcal immunisation
        46
    schedule 45–6
    trips abroad 46, 52
impetigo 210–11
impulsiveness 117
inattention 117
Infacol 29
inguinal hernia 206, 207
inhalers 153, 154
insulin 175, 176, 177
intelligence 109
intussusception 26
itching 213, 214

jaundice 19, **21–2**, 173, 204

joint pains 170, 205
    see also arthritis; cancer; sickle-cell
        disease
Junifen 270
juvenile chronic arthritis *see*
        arthritis
juvenile rheumatoid arthritis *see*
        arthritis

kidney disease 30, 157, 194
kitchen safety 253
Koplik's spots 217

labour and delivery
    at home/in hospital 15–16
    complementary therapies 14
    pain relief 14
    students, presence of 15–16
lactose-free milk preparations 27
laxatives 167, 168
lazy eye 34
learning difficulties 10, 12, 25, 69,
        111, 194, 195
    see also dyslexia
lethargy *see* tiredness
leukaemia 161, 181, 204, **211–13**
    acute 211
    chronic 211
lice infestation 213–15
light, aversion to 193, 203, 220
limping 20, **215–16**
listeria 13
little red book 54
liver disease 22, 51, 104, 170, 194,
        204–6
liver tumours 204
lumbar puncture 222
lung damage 51

magnetic resonance imaging 156
malaria 194
malignant melanoma **158**, 263
massage 14, 78, 83
masturbation 229
measles 44, 45, **50**, **216–19**
meconium 19

medical accident or negligence 143, 145

medical care 133–45

medicine cupboard 269–71

meningitis 18, 32, 39, 45, 50, 173, 193, 194, 203, **219–23**
   bacterial meningitis 220, 221–2
   emergency action 221
   in infancy 221
   meningococcal meningitis 220, 222–3
   symptoms 221
   viral meningitis 219–21

mental handicap 51

mercury allergy 127

methylphenidate 118

midwives 15, 18, 140

migraine 105, 187, 203

milia 22

milk
   cows' milk 95, **97–8**, 104, 107
   goats' milk 99
   sheep's milk 99
   see also formula milks

milk teeth 36, 123, 129

miscarriages 12, 14

moles 158

Mongolian blue spots 22

mood swings 156

morning sickness 14

moro or startle reflex 60

mother and toddler groups 72, 89

mouth ulcers 131

mumps 45, **50**, 175, **223–5**

nappies 82
   disposable 79

nappy rash **35–6**, 37, 56, 82

nasal diphtheria 179

National Childbirth Trust 84, 92

National Health Service Confederation 142

National Health Service (NHS) 128, 129, 133
   complaints procedure 140–1
   dental treatment 128

nausea 156, 157, 202, 204

neck, stiff 161, 193, 203

negative feelings see post-natal depression

Neonatal Unit (NNU) 16, 17, 18

nephroblastoma see Wilm's tumour

nettle sting 104

neuroblastoma 157–8

newborn and first-year babies
   abnormalities and illnesses 22–39
   birth weight 18, 29, 56, 57, **91**
   congenital abnormalities 13, **22–6**
   examination 18–21
   first minutes of life 16
   growth and development 56–64
   overdue babies 18
   premature babies **17–18**, 39, 92, 96

nits see lice infestation

'no', saying 63, 66, 85

nocturnal enuresis see bedwetting

non-accidental injury (NAI) 122

nose bleeds 225–6

nose, blocked and runny 201, 217

nurseries 71–2

nuts 106, 107, 252

ophthalmologist 34

orchidectomy 39

orchidopexy 39

orthodontics 129–30

osteomyelitis 49

osteoporosis 151

osteosarcoma 158–9

otitis externa 183

otitis media 182–3

over-activity 117

overheating 40

paediatric cardiologist 164

paediatricians 15, 18, 67, 138

pain relief 270

palate formation 19

palmar grasp 63

paracetamol preparations 29, 32, 37, 78, 203, 270, 271

paraphimosis 227

parent–child bonding 17
parental health 110
parenthood 87–8
Parents at Work 90
Patient's Charter 142
peak flow test 153, 154
peanuts 106
pemoline 118
penile and foreskin problems 226–9
periodontal disease *see* gum disease
peritonitis 148, 149
permanent dentition 123
pertussis *see* whooping cough
petit mal 188
Peyer's patches 28
pharyngitis 243
Phenergan 270
phenobarbitone 190
Phenoxymethyl penicillin 243
phenylketonuria 21
phenytoin 190
phimosis 226
phlegm 230
physical abuse 110, **122**
pincer grip 63, 65
Piriton 270
plaque 123, 124–5
playgroups 56, **71–2**
playing 56, 66, 67, **70–4**
pneumococcal immunisation 46
pneumococcal infection 237–8
pneumonia 49, 161, 218, **231**
poisoning 262
poliomyelitis (polio) 45, 46, **49**
poliomyelitis vaccine 43, 45
polyps 170
ponds and paddling pools 253–4, 259
port wine stains 22
posseting 101
post-natal depression 31, 56, **88–9**
post-natal support groups 84
practice nurses 135
praise and rewards 85, 117
pregnancy
    alcohol consumption 10
    diet and nutrition 11

drugs, prescribed and illegal
    10–11, 40
exercise 11
folic acid intake 11
genetic screening 13–14, 198–9
German measles 51
health care 54
infections and the unborn baby
    11–13
labour and delivery 14–15
miscarriages 12, 14
smoking **9–10**, 40
termination 13
premature babies **17–18**, 39
    feeding 92, 96
private dental and medical care
    144–5
promethazine 270
pseudoephedrine 147
puberty 57
pure napkin dermatitis 35
pyloric stenosis 30

quality time 72
quinsy 243

rabies 46
rashes **22**, 37, 51, 104, 150, 157, 170,
    193, 203, 221
    purpuric rash 193, **221**
    see also allergies; chickenpox;
        eczema; impetigo; measles;
        meningitis; nappy rash;
        ringworm; scabies; slapped
        cheek syndrome
red eye *see* conjunctivitis; measles
reflexes
    blink reflex 62
    grasp reflex 60
    moro or startle reflex 60
    rooting reflex 61
    stepping reflex 60
    sucking reflex 61
reflux (gastro-oesophageal reflux) 26,
    101–2
Rehidrat 196, 271

relaxation therapy 154–5
Respiratory Distress Syndrome 18
Respiratory Syncytial Virus 28
respiratory tract infections 30, 39–40, 172, 193, **229–33**
resuscitation for children 264–8
retinoblastoma 156–7
Reye's Syndrome 203, 270
rhinitis *see* hay fever
ringworm 233–4
rocking your baby 83
rooting reflex 61
rubella 12, 44, 45, **51**, 162, 173

safety 56, 64, 74
    see also accident prevention
salmon patches 22
salt 100
satellite spots 35
scabies 211, **234–5**
scaly skin *see* ringworm
SCBU (Special Care Baby Unit) 16
school nurses 53, 56, 68
school, physical examinations at 68
school refusal 119, **120**
scoliosis 235–6
screaming fits 26, 29, 82
    see also colic
seborrhoeic eczema 184
septicaemia 18, 45, 49
sexual abuse 110, **121–2**
sexual health 56
sexually transmitted disease 12
sheep's milk 99
shingles 160
shivering 193
shock 256, 257
sibling jealousy 56, 113
sickle-cell disease 198, **236–8**
slapped cheek syndrome 237–9
sleep problems 56, **74–8**
    controlled crying technique 75–6, 78
    early months 74–5
    good sleeping habits, encouraging 78, 83

six months onwards 75
    tackling 75–6
smacking 86
smiling 62
social behaviour
    development 60, 72
    newborn and first-year babies 61–2, 63–4
    second year 65–6
    third year 67
sodium cromoglycate 147
soft drinks 100
soiling 81
solid foods 98–9, 104, 107
sore throats 28, 183, 193, **243–4**
    see also tonsillitis
soya 104
soya milk 105
space-occupying lesions *see* brain tumours
special needs 69–70
    local authority obligations 70
    Statement of Educational Needs 70
speech
    assessments 69
    development 60
    newborn and first-year babies 61, 62, 63
    problems 111–12
    second year 65
    third year 66–7
speech and language therapy 24, 112
spina bifida 11, 19, **23**
spine, curvature of the *see* scoliosis
spleen, damaged 46
splinters 263
sprains and strains (RICE procedure) 263
squint **34–5**, 62
stammering 112
Staphylococcus aureus 210
statementing 70
stepping reflex 60
steroids 147, 151, 153–4, 161, 185, 202

sticky eyes *see* conjunctivitis
Still's disease *see* arthritis
stools 93, 101
   blood in 196–7
   meconium 19
   pale 204
   smelly and greasy 170, 172
stork marks 22
strabismus *see* squint
strangers, wariness of 64, 67
strawberry marks 22
stress 88, 203
stridor 28, 169
stroke 203
sucking 83
sucking reflex 61
Sudden Infant Death Syndrome
   (SIDS) *see* cot death
sugar **99–100**, 125
sunburn 263–4
supervising children 74
suppositories 168
swaddling 83
sweating, excessive 25
sweets 125
syphilis 12

teeth
   braces 129–30
   cleaning 124
   crooked 129
   dental problems 129–32
   dental x-rays 127–8
   fillings 127
   milk teeth 36, 123, 129
   primary dentition 123
   tooth decay 99, **123–6**
   tooth discolouration 126
   toothache 132
   wisdom teeth 123
teething **36–7**, 56, 78, 82, 271
television 72–3
temper tantrums 56, **84–7**
   breath-holding attacks 86–7
   coping with 85–6
temporal lobe epilepsy 188

'terrible twos' 84, 85, 102
testicle problems **239–40**
   cancer 38, 240
   maldescended testicle 38
   retractile testicle 38
   testicular pain 225
   torsion 240
   undescended testicle 19, **37–9**, 68
tetanus 45, 46, **47–8**
thalassaemia 240–2
thalidomide 10, 13
thermometers 78, **192–3**
thirst 176
'three-month colic' 101
thrush 35, 131
thyroid, under-active 21, 182
tired mother/irritable child 31
tiredness 82, 119, 176, 204, 211
   see also diabetes; glandular fever;
     sickle-cell disease; thalassaemia
toddler's diarrhoea 241
toilet training 56, 67, 77, **79–81**
   bedwetting 56, **79–80**, 176
   night-time dryness 79
   soiling 81
tonic clonic *see* grand mal epilepsy
tonsillitis 28, 211, **242–3**
tonsils 217
tooth decay 99, **123–6**
toothache 132
toxoplasmosis 12, 173
toy libraries 71
toys 71
tracheotomy 179
triple or quadruple blood test 14
truancy 120
tuberculosis 45, 46, **51–2**, 194, **231**
tummy pain 26, 148–9, 157, 193,
   204, 221, 245
   see also appendicitis; hepatitis; liver
     problems; mumps
tummy upset/bug 271
   see also gastro-enteritis
twins 117

ultrasound scans 23, 80, 157, 164

umbilical cord 21
umbilical hernia 207
urinary tract infections 27, 30, 80, 193, 203, **244–6**
urine
   blood in the 157, 193
   discoloured 204, 245
   excessive production 176

vaccines *see* immunisation
valproate 190
Varicella-Zoster virus 160
vegan diet 96, **107**
vegetarian diets 96, **106–7**
verrucas and warts 246–7
vision **33–5**, 55, 59–60
   newborn and first-year babies 61, 62, 63
   second year 65
   third year 66
visual disturbances **33–5**, 156, 202, 203
vitamin C 28
vitamin K injections 16
vitamin supplements 95, 97, 104
vomiting 26, 27, **101–2**, 156, 157, 193, 196, 203, 204, 220, 221
   projectile vomiting 30
   see also gastro-enteritis; hepatitis; liver disease; meningitis; reflux

walking *see* crawling/walking
warts *see* verrucas and warts

weaning 56, 94, 95, 96, **98–100**, 102, 105
weight 57
   average birth weight 91
   birth weight 18, 29, 56, 57, **91**
   breast-fed babies 59
   concerns 59
   low birth weight 39
   normal weight gain 91
   overweight children 103–4
   poor weight gain 29–30, 59, 93–4
   routine weighing 59
weight loss 172, 176, 204, 231
   see also coeliac disease; diabetes
wheezing and breathlessness 25, 152, 193, 201, 230, 231
   see also asthma; bronchitis; hay fever; pneumonia
whooping cough 45, **48–9**, **248–50**
Wilm's tumour 157
wind 29, 82
wisdom teeth 123
witch's milk 19
working mothers 72, 89–90

x-rays 127–8, 156, 164

yellow fever 46
yoga 154–5

zinc and castor oil cream 36